Agents and Actions Supplements
Vol. 47

Series Editors
K. Brune, Erlangen
M.J. Parnham, Bonn

Inflammation: Mechanisms and Therapeutics

Edited by
N.S. Doherty
B.M. Weichman
D.W. Morgan
L.A. Marshall

Birkhäuser Verlag
Basel · Boston · Berlin

Editors:

Niall S. Doherty, Ph. D.
Pfizer Central Research
Groton, CT 06340
USA

Barry M. Weichman, Ph. D.
Wyeth-Ayerst Research
Princeton, NJ 08543
USA

Douglas W. Morgan, Ph. D.
Abbott Laboratories
100 Abbott Park, IL 60064
USA

Lisa A. Marshall, Ph. D.
SmithKline Beecham Pharmaceuticals
King of Prussia, PA 19406-0939
USA

A CIP catalogue record for this book is available from the Library of Congress, Washington D.C., USA

Deutsche Bibliothek Cataloging-in-Publication Data
[Agents and actions / Supplements]
Agents and actions. Supplements. - Basel ; Boston ; Berlin :
Birkhäuser.
    Früher Schriftenreihe
    Reihe Supplements zu: Agents and actions
Vol. 47. Inflammation. - 1995
Inflammation : mechanisms and therapeutics / ed. by N. S.
Doherty ...– Basel ; Boston ; Berlin : Birkhäuser, 1995
    (Agents and actions : Supplements ; Vol. 47)
    ISBN-13: 978-3-0348-7345-1

NE: Doherty, Niall S. [Hrsg.]

© 1995 Birkhäuser Verlag, P.O. Box 133, CH-4010 Basel, Switzerland
Softcover reprint of the hardcover 1st edition 1995
Camera-ready copy prepared by the editors and authors
Printed on acid-free paper produced from chlorine-free pulp
Cover design: Heinz Hiltbrunner, Basel

ISBN-13: 978-3-0348-7345-1   e-ISBN-13: 978-3-0348-7343-7
DOI: 10.1007/978-3-0348-7343-7

Contents

Workshop Sessions

Preface

The Seventh International Conference of the Inflammation Research Association, entitled "Inflammation, Mechanisms and Therapeutics" was held on September 25-29, 1994 in White Haven, Pennsylvania. The major focus of this series of conferences is the multidisciplinary investigation of inflammation and the discovery of novel therapeutic approaches to inflammatory diseases. It was therefore particularly gratifying that the list of attendees included scientists of diverse backgrounds – preclinical biology, synthetic and theoretical chemistry, biotechnology and clinical research. The Conference was characterized by a very high degree of participation in the scientific debate by attendees, a large proportion of whom presented at poster sessions, poster discussions and workshops, and by the many opportunities for informal discussion provided by the organizers. This volume captures much of the excitement and enthusiasm of the Conference and should be a valuable resource for scientists in the field.

Niall S. Doherty
Barry M. Weichman
Douglas W. Morgan
Lisa A. Marshall

Acknowledgments

The manuscripts contained in this volume are based on material presented at the Seventh International Conference of the Inflammation Research Association held in White Haven, Pennsylvania, on September 25-29, 1994.

We would like to thank the speakers and session chairpersons for their contributions to the Conference and these Proceedings.

The following individuals played indispensable roles in the organization and running of the Conference and are responsible for making it such a success:

PLANNING
Niall S. Doherty
Barry M. Weichman
Douglas Morgan
D. Euan MacIntyre

ADVERTISING
Dennis Roland

AUDIO-VISUAL
Thomas J. Carty, Chairperson
John Lee, Co-Chairperson
John Barberia
Ronald Laliberte
Amy Roshak
Linne Svensson

FINANCE
D. Euan MacIntyre

POSTER SESSION/ABSTRACT BOOK
Joanne Uhl, Chairperson
Loran Killar
Lisa Marshall
John Lee

PUBLICATIONS
Niall S. Doherty
Barry Weichman
Douglas Morgan
Lisa Marshall

REGISTRAR
Joan M. Chapdelaine

SCIENTIFIC PROGRAM
Barry M. Weichman, Chairperson
Robert J. Smith
Christopher H. Evans
Dennis Roland
Guy Schiehser
Steven Gilman
Alison Badger
L. Gordon Letts
Don Anderson

POSTER DISCUSSION
Nigel Boughton-Smith
Gerald DeVries
Robert Jacobs
Mark Miller

SCHOLARSHIP
Janet Kerr, Chairperson
Richard Carlson
Richard Harris
Loran Killar
Ivan Otterness
Ann Welton
John Young

SITE COORDINATION
Hui-Lian Liauw
Marcia L. Bliven
Deborah A. Wolff

TRAVEL ARRANGEMENTS
Alan J. Main

SOCIAL EVENTS
Robbin Breslow, Chairperson
Lynn Brophy

WORKSHOP SESSIONS
Douglas Morgan, Co-Chairperson
Lisa Marshall, Co-Chairperson
Alejandro Aruffo
Mary Barnette
Michael DiMartino
Francis Dumont
Keith Glaser
David Grass
Richard Griffiths
Don Griswold
John Lackie
Carmine Lanni
Dave Manning
Bruce Miller
Eugene Mochan
Karl Mollison
S. N. S. Murthy
Elizabeth O'Bryne
Adrian Payne
William Selig

The generous financial support of the following companies is greatly appreciated:

Abbott Laboratories
Biomol Research
Burroughs Wellcome Co.
Ciba Pharmaceuticals
DuPont Merck Pharmaceutical Co.
Genentech, Inc.
Hoffmann-LaRoche, Inc.
Janssen Research Foundation
3M Pharmaceuticals
Merck Frosst Canada
Merck Research Laboratories
Pfizer Inc, Central Research Division

Perseptive Diagnostics
Pharmakon Research International
Schering-Plough Research Institute
SmithKline Beecham Pharmaceuticals
Sterling Winthrop, Inc.
Syntex, Inc.
Wyeth-Ayerst Research
Yamanouchi UK

Sincere appreciation is extended to the following Corporations for their additional contribution:

Abbott Laboratories ....Registration folders

CIBA Pharmaceuticals ....Signs

Merck Research Laboratories...Registration materials

Pfizer Inc, Central Research Division ....Program and miscellaneous printed materials

Pharmakon Research International, Inc.................................Name tags / registration

SmithKline Beecham Pharmaceuticals ....Abstract booklet

Wyeth-Ayerst Research ....Service awards

AAS 47
Inflammation:
Mechanisms and Therapeutics
© 1995 Birkhäuser Verlag Basel

THE PATHOGENESIS OF RHEUMATOID ARTHRITIS AND THE DEVELOPMENT OF THERAPEUTIC STRATEGIES FOR THE CLINICAL INVESTIGATION OF BIOLOGICS

Professor Gabriel S Panayi ScD, MD, FRCP.
Arthritis and Rheumatism Council
Professor of Rheumatology
Guy's Hospital, London, England

SUMMARY: This review discusses current concepts of the pathogenesis of rheumatoid arthritis. It is proposed that RA is a T cell mediated disease following which a large number of subsequent inflammatory events are unleashed. Many of the pathogenetic steps are targets for new therapies including biologics. Laboratory, clinical and radiological methods of assessing disease activity are sufficiently sensitive and reproducible to permit their use in multicentre studies capable of detecting a biologic with disease modifying activity. The clinical assessment of the efficacy and toxicity of biologics poses unique problems. These have been illustrated by the example of 3 monoclonal antibodies directed against ICAM-1, CD4 and TNFα. The main role of most biologics may be to pinpoint important therapeutic targets which can be attacked by more easily administered and less costly xenobiotic drugs.

INTRODUCTION

The present is a pivotal time for the development of new therapies for the treatment of rheumatoid arthritis (RA). Our understanding of the pathogenesis of the disease is now firmly grounded in cellular and molecular concepts, we have begun to develop clinically useful prognostic factors and we can monitor disease activity more effectively, reproducibly and economically. An additional and critical factor for the development of therapeutic strategies has been the establishment of academic rheumatology centres familiar with the laboratory as well as with the clinical aspects of RA.

PATHOGENESIS OF RHEUMATOID ARTHRITIS

The current concepts of the pathogenesis of RA are based on immunogenetic, immunohistological and functional studies.

Immunogenetics of RA RA is strongly associated, in most populations studied, with certain subtypes of the β chain of HLA-DR4. These subtypes are dependent on polymorphisms of the third hypervariable region (HVR III) of the β chain. The HVR III of HLA-DR1 and of HLA-DR10 show sequence similarities to the disease-associated subtypes of HLA-DR4 (Table 1).

Table 1   Summary of HLA-DRß1 allelic associations with rheumatoid arthritis together with third hypervariable region pentapeptide sequences[1]

Serological Specificity	Allele HLA-DRb1	Previous equivalent	HVR3 (70-74) pentapeptide[a]	Association with RA
DR4	0401	Dw4	QKRAA	Positive
DR4	0404	Dw14.1	QRRAA	Positive
DR4	0405	Dw15	QRRAA	Positive
DR4	0408	Dw14.2	QRRAA	Positive
DR1	0101	Dw1	QRRAA	Positive
DRw14	1402	Dw16	QRRAA	Positive
DRw10	1001	-	RRRAA	Positive
DR4	0402	Dw10	<u>DER</u>AA	Negative
DR4	0403	Dw13.1	QRRA<u>E</u>	Negative
DR4	0407	Dw13.2	QRRA<u>E</u>	Negative
DR2(w15)	1501	Dw2	<u>D</u>RRAA	Negative
DR5(w11)	1101	Dw5	<u>D</u>RRAA	Negative
DR4	0406	DwKT2	QRRA<u>E</u>	Unknown[b]
DR4	0409	-	QKRAA	Unknown

[a]Amino acid sequences are given in single-letter code. Underlining indicates a non-conservative substitution compared to the QRRAA template.
[b]Indicates insufficient population data exist to estimate RA association.

This similarity is central to the "shared epitope hypothesis" (10) although the use of the

---

[1]   Official WHO nomenclature is given for each allele e.g. HLA-DRß1*0401 refers to the HLA-DRß1 allele associated with the Dw4 HLA-D specificity.

term "epitope" seems inappropriate in this context. Since the HVR III is a critical component in the formation of the groove which binds antigenic peptides for their presentation to the T cell receptor of responding T cells, the HLA association with RA suggests that appropriate antigenic peptides may be involved in the initiation and perpetuation of the disease. An excess of particular TCR Vβ families within the rheumatoid joint has been found but there is no general consensus on this finding. The failure to find a particular TCR to be commonly expressed in the joint of patients with RA suggests that disease-causing T cells are probably present in low frequency.

Antigens in RA   The nature of the antigens involved in the aetiopathogenesis of RA is still unknown. Several candidate antigens have been proposed. They include type II collagen, found uniquely in articular cartilage, cartilage proteoglycan and heat shock proteins. However, none of them has become generally accepted in the way in which, for example, the acetylcholine receptor has become accepted as the autoantigenic target in myasthenia gravis. The involvement of type II collagen (CII) is based mainly on serological evidence as it has proved extremely difficult to stimulate human T cells with native CII. Even so, only a minority of patients have high titres of anti-CII antibodies which are linked to HLA-DR7 and not to HLA-DR4 (15). Although CII is found in nasal, aural and tracheal cartilages, these sites are not involved in RA raising doubts as to the presence of CII autoimmunity. Little work has been done on the autoantigenic role of cartilage proteoglycan but it is probably of greater pathogenetic role in ankylosing spondylitis. There are several problems with the role of heat shock proteins (HSP) as antigens in RA which limitation of space prevents full discussion. The 2 major criticisms are: lack of tissue specificity and the low frequency of T cells responding to 65KD HSP, which is proposed as the main candidate, found in RA synovial fluid (8). Clearly a new approach is required and we have used reverse genetics in our search for the rheumatoid autoantigen.

Chondrocyte autoimmunity in RA   Articular cartilage contains cells unique in structure, function and secretory capacity: the chondrocytes. Thus, RA could be viewed as an organ-specific disease with the autoimmune attack directed against chondrocyte specific structures or products. Indeed, the proposal that type II collagen or cartilage proteoglycan are rheumatoid autoantigens are aspects of this hypothesis. More recently, interest has been aroused in chondrocyte cell membrane structures as possible autoantigens. Clinical support for the organ specificity of RA is provided by the observation that total condylar resection, as happens during total knee joint replacement, leads to a melting away of the synovitis despite continuing disease activity elsewhere (18). In this operation the synovium is not removed, but does of course remain fully accessible to blood borne cells and factors, such as immune complexes. By contrast, total synovectomy of a knee joint, which was a frequent operation until some years ago, fell into disrepute because remission of synovitis was poor and short lived. Yet RA has up to now been classified in the group of organ non-specific connective tissue diseases since the classical autoantibody found in RA sera, "rheumatoid" factor, is an antiglobulin which does not recognise cellular antigens.

In our approach to chondrocyte autoimmunity in RA, we have shown that a high proportion of rheumatoid sera have antibodies directed against components of a human articular chondrocyte or chondrosarcoma extract. A prominent component is an approximately 65kD protein. Using the procedure outlined in Fig. 1, we have constructed an immunoaffinity column by cutting out the 65kD band from an SDS-PAGE gel slab, homogenising it, constructing a column, passing a pool of RA sera through it and eluting from it high titre antibodies which react strongly with the 65kD chondrocyte/chondrosarcoma-antigen.

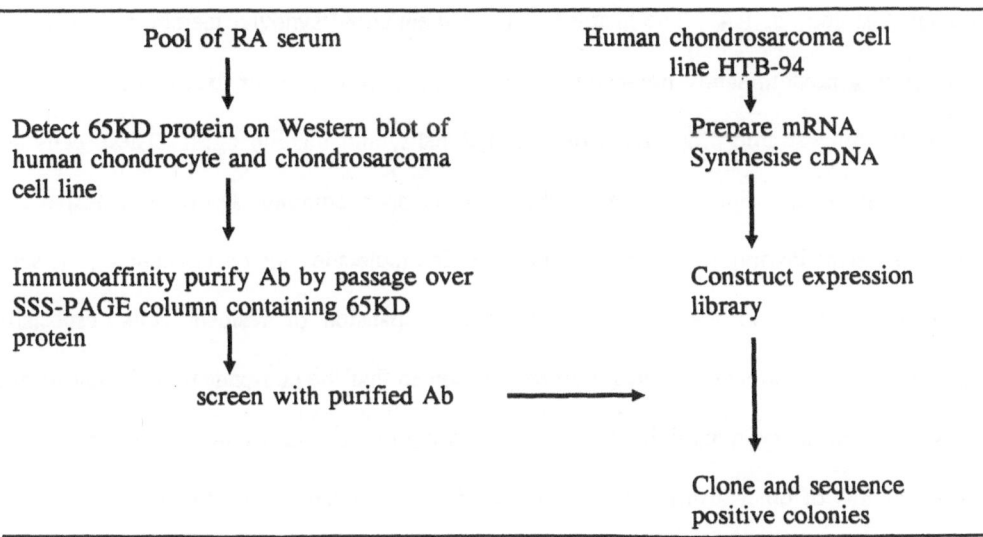

Figure 1. Flow diagram showing the procedure used to clone and sequence the gene coding for a chondrocyte autoantigen of relevance to the pathogenesis of rheumatoid arthritis.

A λ Zap chondrosarcoma cDNA expression library was screened with the immunopurified RA serum and positive phage plaques were picked. Following the tertiary screen an *in vivo* excision method was used to isolate the double-stranded cloned DNA insert of interest. The sequence was unique not being found in the Genbank or EMBL databases. The gene was only expressed in the chondrosarcoma line and not in tissues such as liver, spleen or kidney and not B, T or macrophage cell lines (data not shown). Of course, much work remains to be done with this system but these findings suggest to me that we may, in the near future, be in a position to develop immunotherapy protocols specific for RA using disease-specific autoantigens or reagents derived from them.

Immunohistology of RA   The histology of the rheumatoid synovial membrane (SM) may vary from a predominantly non-cellular collagenous appearance, or to a mononuclear cell infiltrate with variable proportions of T and B cells, and macrophages.   These cells are haematogenous in origin and their entry depends on a complex series of adhesive and migratory steps involving endothelial cells, adhesion molecules and chemotactic agents such as IL-8, MCP-1 and RANTES.   There is an expansion of resident cells, especially endothelial cells and synoviocytes, by proliferation so that the consequent angiogenesis and hyperplasia of the synovial lining layer are the only truly quantitative distinguishing features from the SM of other arthritides.   Angiogenesis is promoted by several factors including TNFα, IL-8 and an as yet uncharacterised vascular endothelial growth factor (16).   Hence, the inhibition of angiogenesis is an attractive therapeutic target.   The synovial lining contains two cell populations with different origins and functions.   Type A cells are bone marrow derived mature monocyte/macrophages which are constantly replaced via the circulation. Type B cells are fibroblast-like cells.   An increase in the number of cells which occupy the synovial lining layer is a striking observation in RA and may be unique to this disease.

The T cells are characteristically arranged in perivascular aggregates.   The cells are predominantly of the CD4+ CD45RO+ phenotype (21).   They have many of the features of activated T cells (Table 2).

Table 2.   Features characteristic of activation found on rheumatoid synovial T cells

ACTIVATION MARKERS:	Function:
CD69	Very early marker
HLA-DR	Intermediate marker
VLA-1	Very late marker
G0 of the cell cycle	
Spontaneous synthesis of: interleukin 6 interferon γ interleukin 2 interleukin 10	
Increased adhesion to endothelial cells	Increased migration into joint
Stimulated IL-1 and TNFα production by monocytes through cell-to-cell contact	Contribution to pathogenesis

However, their exact contribution to the pathogenesis of RA is still not clear (see below). B cells may be found as isolated collections of cells distributed within the SM or as classical lymphoid follicles in up to one third of SM examined. These focal lymphoid aggregates are found more frequently in the SM specimens obtained at the time of surgery from patients with advanced disease compared to synovial biopsies obtained from patients at the time of RA diagnosis. The plasma cells derived from them secrete rheumatoid factors, but up to 90% of them in some membranes secrete immunoglobulins whose antigenic specificities are unknown (5). It may be that some of these antibodies are directed against putative chondrocyte autoantigens, and indeed, this possibility has motivated the experiments described above and illustrated in Fig. 1. All of the monocyte/macrophage series are enriched in the RA SM both in the lining and the sub-lining regions. There are increased numbers of inflammatory monocytes as well as mature macrophages which contribute to inflammation and joint destruction by releasing a number of cytokines as well as enzymes such as collagenase. Of particular relevance is the enrichment of antigen-presenting dendritic cells as these would be contributing to ongoing inflammation by the continuous presentation of autoantigenic peptides to disease specific T cells (22).

Immunohistology has been used to detect the presence of lymphokines, cytokines and growth factors of relevance to inflammation. A vast number of them have been found (Table 3).

Table 3   The lymphokines, cytokines and growth factors
             found in rheumatoid synovium

Lymphokines:
             Interleukins -2, -6, -8, -10
             Interferon γ

Cytokines:
             Interleukin 1α and 1β
             Tumor necrosis factor α
             Chemokines: RANTES, MCP-1, MIP-1α and 1β

Growth factors
             Platelet derived growth factor
             GM-CSF
             Vascular endothelial growth factor
             Transforming growth factor β

The presence of the corresponding mRNA has also been found by techniques such as in situ hybridisation, northern blot hybridisation and the reverse transcriptase polymerase chain reaction (RT-PCR). The presence of all the pro-inflammatory mediators must be placed in the context of an array of anti-inflammatory factors such as TGFß, IL-10, IL-1ra and soluble TNFα receptors, for example, but their quantity is clearly insufficient to control the inflammatory process. Increasing their concentration is a therapeutic aim which is being actively pursued at present and the results of controlled trials are eagerly awaited.

The presence of enzymes within the RA SM, of crucial importance for joint damage, will not be reviewed here.

Immune function in RA   The great obstacle to our understanding of the pathogenesis of RA is the lack of an aetiological agent which triggers and maintains the disease (see above). It is therefore impossible to unravel the immunological consequences of the trigger itself from the adaptive or reactive responses of the host. The classical T cell lymphokines (interleukin 2 and interferon γ) have proved difficult to demonstrate as being spontaneously produced within the rheumatoid joint. Since antigen specific T cells are found in low frequency in a lesion driven by that antigen, then IL-2 and IFNγ may not have to be present in high concentration in order to drive the disease (20). Interleukin 10 (IL-10) is produced in significant amounts in the joint both by T cells and other cells. The presence of this TH2 lymphokine suggests that an adaptive host response is being made but which is incapable of adequately suppressing immune-mediated inflammation (11). There is additional evidence for such an adaptive response in the high levels of circulating and local interleukin 1 receptor antagonist (IL-1ra), and soluble TNFα p55 and p75 receptors.

The production of many pro-inflammatory cytokines and growth factors from macrophages, synoviocytes and endothelial cells with the paucity of T cell lymphokines has suggested to some investigators that, after a certain stage in the natural history of RA, the disease may be T cell independent. This may be termed the "mesenchymal hypothesis". It is difficult to reconcile this concept with the oft repeated clinical observation that synovitis remits in a knee joint which has undergone total joint replacement despite ongoing inflammation in other joints (see above).

PROGNOSTIC FACTORS IN RA

The development of prognostic factors in RA would permit the early and aggressive treatment of patients who are likely to develop joint destruction, pain, loss of function and to experience a poor quality of life while reserving milder treatment for patients with a better prognosis. We are far from this goal. The following have been proposed as prognostic markers: HLA-DR4, RF and sulphoxidation status.

In northern European populations, HLA-DR4 is associated with a poor prognosis. In other populations, however, the prevalence of HLA-DR4, and of other members of the "shared epitope" in general, is lower. This is the situation in the Greek population, for example. In the Greeks, RA is milder than in northern Europeans. Of great interest is the fact that there is no difference in severity of RA between DR4+ and DR4- RA in Greeks (4). This lack of severity may be due to environmental factors although the involvement of unknown genes, which modulate disease expression, cannot be excluded. Hence, HLA-DR4 itself cannot be indiscriminately used as a severity factor. In addition, there is evidence that homozygosity for HLA-DR4 is associated with severe disease especially Felty's syndrome (17).

Many studies have shown that high titres of RF are associated with more severe RA both in terms of joint erosion as well as extra-articular features. There are, again, population differences since extra-articular manifestations are rare in Greeks although high titres of RF are found as in northern Europe.

Previous studies have shown that poor sulphoxidation of acetylcysteine is associated with RA (7). More recently, poor sulphoxidation has been proposed as a poor prognostic marker but this has not been universally verified.

Thus, patients who possess one of the DR4β1 "shared epitopes" or a high titre of IgM RF at or soon after the onset of RA will probably have a poor prognosis (9). However, that prognosis cannot, at present, be directly translated into the number of orthopaedic operations, the quality of life or the economic cost of the disease after 5, 10 or 15 years duration. Such nomograms are urgently needed.

DISEASE MONITORING IN RA

The development of effective therapies will be difficult to assess if the instruments available for monitoring different aspects of disease activity in RA are crude, insensitive and poorly reproducible. There are 3 main ways of monitoring disease activity and hence of outcome following drug therapy: clinical, laboratory and radiologic.

Clinical assessment   Clinical assessment remains the mainstay of drug evaluation. The simplified core set of data, agreed to by the ACR, EULAR and the WHO are a very welcome and long delayed step. They are an economical, reproducible and internationally agreed and validated set of clinical disease activity criteria (23). It is to be hoped that properly conducted trials, wherever carried out, based on these criteria, will be acceptable for registration by different national and supranational drug agencies wherever carried out. Other measures which are being developed, but are not yet in general use, include quality of life outcome and health economic costs of treatment. Quality of life outcomes pose problems for drug development. Since quality of life can only be truly judged in the long term, it will be difficult if not impossible to meaningfully include such measures in drug trials which are, of necessity, short term. From the health economic point of view two issues need to be considered. First, treatment which significantly abolishes pain and/or the systemic features of RA (malaise, loss of weight) has clinical utility and deserves to be in the pharmacopoeia but may not necessarily result in significant economic benefits. Second, treatment which produces prolonged remission of disease deserves licensing even if each "course" of treatment carries a high cost. It should not be forgotten that RA not only produces the well known joint problems but also significantly reduces life expectancy to a comparable extent as acknowledged serious diseases such as coronary artery disease or Hodgkin's disease. Patients with chronic disease, such as RA, must not be sacrificed on the altar of economic necessity.

<u>Laboratory assessment</u>   Laboratory measures of disease activity can be broadly divided into those which attempt to measure cartilage and bone damage and those which measure the acute phase response. The former have not yet been developed sufficiently for routine use. As a consequence, the acute phase response is used as a surrogate marker for joint damage. Cytokines, such as IL-1, TNFα, IL-6 and LIF, released from the inflamed joint, stimulate hepatocytes to increased synthesis and secretion of a number of proteins. The concentration of cytokines is thought to be related to the degree of inflammation and hence of eventual joint destruction. The concentration of acute phase proteins collectively or singly reflect the degree of inflammation. The two commonest measures are the C-reactive protein (CRP) and the erythrocyte sedimentation rate (ESR). Several studies have shown that the height of the acute phase response correlates with the degree of eventual radiological joint damage especially if the acute phase response is quantified as the product of the ESR or CRP with time (24). Hence, measure of the CRP and/or ESR must be included in any clinical trial. Some investigators prefer the CRP over the ESR but there is no general consensus over this; CRP has the advantage of a much greater range over which it can be modulated than ESR, while the latter is more easily measured in all laboratories.

<u>Radiological assessment</u>   This is considered by many to be the gold standard by which to measure the long term efficacy of new or established drugs in RA. The disadvantage of this approach is that studies would take a long time and would be expensive. Furthermore, placebo controlled studies of such a duration (1 year or more) cannot be ethically justified. Such studies should be undertaken only after preliminary studies have shown that the drug under investigation suppresses synovitis, improves subjective measures of disease activity and lowers the acute phase response. Several existing drugs, such as sulphasalazine, cyclophosphamide and gold, have been shown, in prospective controlled studies lasting 1 year, to retard radiological progression.

Active studies are in progress which attempt to evaluate newer forms of radiological assessment for the measurement of joint damage such as DEXA scans of the hands and magnetic resonance imaging. Long term studies are not yet available - the former seems most promising. The latter is currently too expensive for routine use.

New drugs must therefore be shown to be symptomatically effective, with normalisation of laboratory measures of inflammation and/or tissue destruction in the short term, with retardation or cessation of radiological joint damage in the long term.

THE EVALUATION OF BIOLOGICS IN RHEUMATOID ARTHRITIS

Having established the pathogenetic and clinical basis of RA, one can now review the evaluation of biologics in RA. A large number of biologics have been, are being and will be evaluated for their potential role as effective and tolerated therapies for the treatment of RA and a list is given in Table 4.

Table 4   Biologics which have been and are being evaluated as potential therapies in RA

1.	Monoclonal/chimaeric/humanised Abs:	
	(a) to T cells:	CD7, IL-2R, CD5-PLUS (CD5 ricin), CD3, CD4, CDW62 (CAMPATH-1H)
	(b) to adhesion molecules:	ICAM-1
	(c) to cytokines:	TNFα
2.	Soluble inhibitors/receptors:	
	IL-1ra, sTNFR p55 and p75 sIL-1R type I and II sCR1	
3.	Cytokines and toxin	
	IL2-DAB toxin	

Some, such as anti-CD7 antibodies, are no longer under active consideration as preliminary studies showed no therapeutic benefit whatsoever. Others, such as CD5 PLUS and IL-2DAB, have had their further development in RA temporarily suspended. Others, such as antibodies to CD4, ICAM-1 and to TNFα, soluble interleukin 1 receptor antagonist and soluble TNFα receptors, are under active investigation at present. It would obviously be an impossible task in the space allotted to me to review all these developments. Consequently, I shall confine myself to the discussion of general principles learnt in some 7 years of personal involvement in this field.

What are the aims of therapy with biologics?

Most biologics have exquisite specificity because they are antibodies, soluble receptors or receptor antagonists. The discovery of clinical efficacy is *prima facie* evidence that the targets, against which biologics are directed, are of relevance to the pathogenesis of RA. Hence, the first aim in evaluating any new biologic is to determine whether it has any effect on rheumatoid disease activity (Fig. 2).

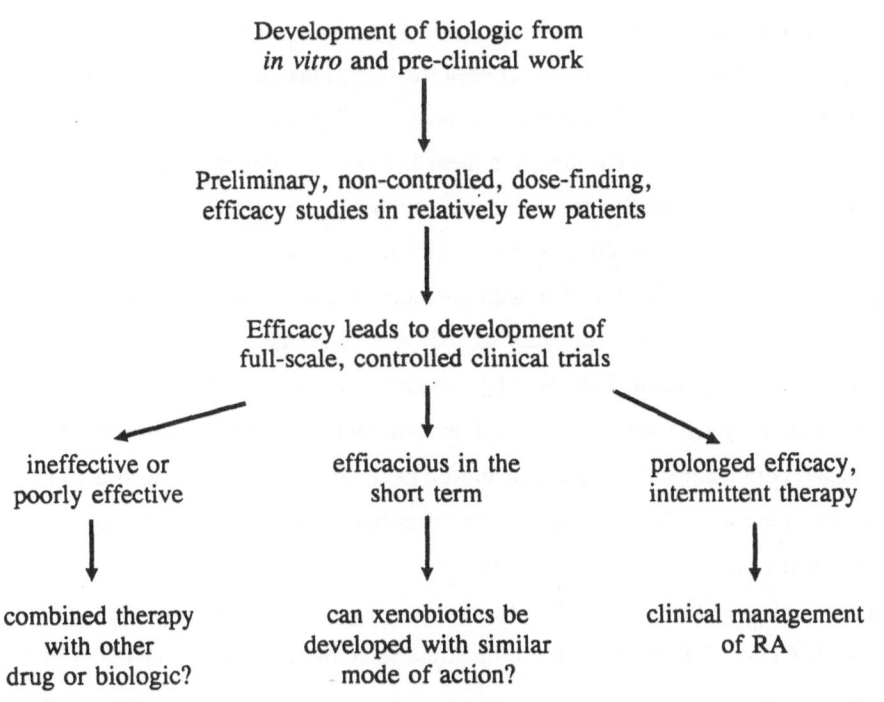

Figure 2.   The developmental aims of biologic therapy

An affirmative answer then leads to the next question. Can this therapy be used for the clinical management of RA or can it be substituted in the long term by an appropriately synthesised xenobiotic? The recently conducted open study of anti-TNFα antibody (chimaeric Ca2, Centocor) has shown considerable promise in the short term. Several existing xenobiotics apparently have anti-TNFα activity (Tenidap (Pfizer) inhibits its production, oxpentyfylline (Hoechst) inhibits its action, and yet others are under development. Whether a biologic or a xenobiotic will be used in anti-TNFα therapy will therefore be determined in the long run by the usual considerations of cost (including cost of administration), efficacy and toxicity. Anti-TNFα therapy may be short lived and treatment will therefore have to be given over years. An alternative scenario is that treatment with a biologic could lead to a prolonged remission of disease during which no further treatment is required. An example from animal work is the so-called "infectious tolerance" induced by the administration of anti-CD4 monoclonal antibody (1). Such therapy seems unlikely to be superseded by the use of xenobiotics. Intermittent therapy, if unaccompanied by toxic side-effects, would be perfectly acceptable for the clinical management of RA if the intervals between treatments are sufficiently long to make the cost of treatment reasonable. Finally, there is the possibility that combined therapy could achieve prolonged remission; so far such treatment has been in animal models in which collagen arthritis was arrested by combined treatment with anti-TNFα and anti-CD4 antibodies (25). Of course, such therapy could be a combination of a biologic with a xenobiotic; a theoretical combination could be anti-TNFα with methotrexate or cyclosporin A. However, such combination therapy must be approached with extreme caution as unacceptable and unpredictable drug interactions may be encountered. Thus, the combination of anti-CD4 antibody therapy with methotrexate led to extremely low numbers of CD4+ T cells for prolonged periods of time (2 years or more)(19) unlike our study when anti-CD4 was given alone in which the CD4 lymphopenia was transient (lasting less than 6 months) and not as severe (Choy and Panayi, unpublished).

The story of three therapies. I shall review the experience with antibodies directed against ICAM-1, CD4 and TNFα in order to illustrate some of the problems involved in developing a biologic therapy for RA.

(a)   Anti-ICAM-1 therapy

ICAM-1 is found on lymphoid cells whilst its counter-receptor LFA-1 is found not only on lymphoid cells but also on endothelial cells. It is involved in immune reactions and in the adhesion to and migration through endothelial cells by T lymphocytes. Antibodies to ICAM-1 inhibit T cell mediated immune reactions both *in vivo* and *in vitro* and will inhibit T cell adhesion to human umbilical vein endothelial cells *in vitro*. It is, consequently, an important therapeutic target in RA in which T cell migration into and cell-mediated immune reactions within the synovium are thought to be such prominent events.

In the development of antibody therapy directed against ICAM-1 (BIRR1), the problem had to be faced that with the widespread expression of the molecule, achieving effective serum concentrations might require relatively large amounts of antibody. A dose sufficient to give free antibody in the circulation was established in renal allograft recipients. It was established that a loading dose of 120 mg followed by 40 mg daily of antibody over 5 days achieved measurable serum concentrations in all patients. Experiments showed that $\geq$ $10\mu g/ml$ BIRR1 caused 100% inhibition of LFA-1/ICAM-1 dependent adhesive interactions *in vitro*. On the basis of these 2 results, an open, uncontrolled study of BIRR1 was executed (12). Administration produced a lymphocytosis and suppression of delayed cutaneous hypersensitivity reactions to recall antigens - outcomes which were predicted from the known activities of ICAM-1. More importantly, the antibody infusion led to clinical and laboratory improvements in disease activity in a significant proportion of the patients in whom serum concentration of BIRR1 exceeded 10 $\mu g/mg$. Interestingly, some of these had prolonged improvements in their disease lasting several weeks. This prolonged clinical effect suggests that anti-ICAM-1 therapy may induce prolonged perturbations in immune responses which may be akin to tolerance induction. Although this would be advantageous from the point of view of the control of RA, it might be disadvantageous in that infections or other complications might arise; long term toxicity and efficacy studies are needed to exclude this possibility.

Thus, a rational approach based on the known involvement of ICAM-1 in immune mechanisms of relevance to the pathogenesis of RA, the use of a dose of antibody sufficient to saturate cell-bound and cell-free ICAM-1 molecules, and the execution of a well planned but open clinical trial has opened the way to large, controlled studies which will allow a proper assessment of the efficacy and tolerability of this therapy.

(b)   Anti-CD4 antibody therapy

The CD4 molecule is found on T helper lymphocytes, some macrophages and the microglia of the central nervous system. It is involved in immune reactions by acting as an accessory molecule interacting with a non polymorphic residue on the HLA-DRB1 chain. Monoclonal antibodies directed against CD4 inhibit cell-mediated reactions *in vitro* and *in vivo*, prevent allograft rejection, improve experimental arthritis in animals, and can induce "infectious tolerance". Part of the mechanism of action is due to death of the reacting T cell by apoptosis. In our own work, we found that $\geq$ 10 μg/ml of cM-T412 was required *in vitro* to suppress T cell stimulation.

The development of anti-CD4 therapy in RA is marked, unlike that for anti-ICAM-1, by a more haphazard or empirical approach whether mouse or chimaeric antibodies were used. We decided to use a more step-by-step approach since biologics may have unexpected therapeutic and toxic side effects. We showed that 50mg intravenously of cM-T412, a chimaeric anti-CD4 antibody (Centocor), produced transient CD4 lymphopenia but had no effect on RA disease activity (3). A similar dose was then used weekly on 4 occasions, but apart from a more prolonged CD4 lymphopenia, there was again, no effect on RA disease activity. It therefore came as no surprise when Moreland *et al* showed in a large, placebo-controlled study that 50mg cM-T412 given monthly produced no clinical benefit (19). It is wrong to conclude from this study, as some will undoubtedly do, that cM-T412 is without therapeutic benefit in RA. The correct conclusion from the study is that an inadequate dose was used.

The next step in our development programme for cM-T412 was to infuse 50 mg daily on 5 consecutive days (3). Patients were then randomised to 2 different regimes. In the "maintenance" regime they received 50 mg weekly for 5 weeks. In the "retreatment" regime they received 50 mg daily for 5 days starting at week 4. The results were essentially the same and will be reviewed as one study. Following this therapy, CD4 lymphopenia was more prolonged. Patients with the lymphopenia beyond 6 months were those taking oral maintenance prednisolone up to 7.5 mg daily. This finding emphasised the unexpected drug interactions possible with biologics (see above for methotrexate/cM-T412 interactions and extremely prolonged CD4 lymphopenia). Following this dosing regimen we saw clinical benefit for the first time in that 3 patients were in remission for at least 9 months after a single course of therapy.

It may be objected that this was an open study and that any clinical benefits seen should be accepted with extreme caution. While true, the following points should be borne in mind. First, placebo effects in our group are small since no improvements were seen with the first

2 dosing regimens or in our previous studies with anti-CD7 antibody (14). Second, clinical improvement correlated with the percentage of CD4 T cells in SF fluids coated with cM-T412 after the fifth dose; 2 of the 3 patients with prolonged improvement had the highest percentage coating of SF CD4 T cells being greater than 75 per cent. SF from patients who did not respond to cM-T412 had CD4 T cells with low or absent antibody coating. Third, cM-T412 SF concentrations were extremely variable with most patients showing little or no antibody in the SF. Free serum cM-T412 was present only transiently confirming that insufficient antibody had been infused.

These studies, which we and others have carried out with cM-T412 in RA, suggest that anti-CD4 antibodies should not be used at present in combination with disease modifying drugs and that the correct dose and dosing regimen have still not been arrived at. In my opinion, it is wrong to discontinue development with this or similar antibodies until these avenues have been fully explored. The story of anti-CD4 therapy is in stark contrast to that for anti-ICAM-1 in which an adequate dose of antibody was found before the therapeutic trial was embarked upon.

(c)   Anti-TNFα antibody therapy

In contrast to CD4 and ICAM-1, which are present on high concentration on cell surfaces and which are also found in soluble form in biologic fluids, TNFα is an induced mediator of inflammation. It is not normally found in the body and its concentration is low after induction although it is biologically very potent. It is believed to play an important role in mediating the inflammatory and joint damaging events within the rheumatoid joint. Anti-TNFα antibodies have been shown to ameliorate inflammation in collagen induced arthritis (2) while mice transgenic for human TNFα spontaneously develop an inflammatory arthritis which is suppressed by anti-TNFα (13). For these reasons, anti-TNFα therapy has been proposed for RA.

An open, uncontrolled study of an anti-TNFα antibody (cA2, Centocor) has shown clinical benefit (6). The dose of antibody used was approximately 1.4g given in one or two divided doses. This should be compared with the 250 mg of cM-T412 given over 5 days or the 280 mg of BIRR1 given over 5 days. The disproportionality of these doses becomes even more apparent when the relative concentration of the various target molecules is considered. Two controlled studies of anti-TNFα therapy are now under way; one using the cA2 (Centocor) and the other the CDP-571 (Celltech) antibody.

These 3 studies have shown 3 distinct differences in approach in developing a biologic therapy for the treatment of RA. It is my contention that the lessons learnt from them (Table 5) should considerably shorten clinical testing time and hence costs. It should be particularly noted that these developmental studies were all carried out as open-label protocols. Furthermore, the number of centres participating in these open studies should be kept to a minimum and restricted to those with the appropriate clinical as well as immunological expertise.

Table 5   Guidelines for developing an antibody based therapy for RA

1.   Quantity and tissue distributions of target molecule.
2.   Develop *in vitro* and, if possible, animal data on effective serum concentration.
3.   Open-label studies in patients with RA to:
     (a)   establish effective dose and dosing regimen for adequate serum and joint
           concentrations;
     (b)   tolerability and safety profile;
     (c)   efficacy.
4.   Institute controlled studies using dose and dosing regimen previously determined
     in (3,a) above.

ACKNOWLEDGEMENTS

I would like to thank my colleagues Drs Jerry S Lanchbury, Ghada Yanni, Ernest Choy, Paul Emery, David Scott and Ms Lesley Forrest for helpful advice and criticism. Experimental work in my laboratory has been funded by the Arthritis and Rheumatism Council and a "BRIDGE" contract by the European Community. I thank Sue Dorward and Valerie Heard for typing the manuscript.

REFERENCES

1. Benjamin RJ, Qin Shixin , Wise MP, Cobbold SP, Waldmann H. Mechanisms of monoclonal antibody-facilitated tolerance induction: a possible role for the CD4 (L3T4) and CD11a (LFA-1) molecules in self-non-self discrimination. Eur J Immunol 1988; 18:1079-1088.

2. Brennan FM, Maini RN, Feldmann M. TNF alpha - a pivotal role in rheumatoid arthritis? Brit J Rheumatol 1992; 31:293-298.

3. Choy EHS, Chikanza IC, Kingsley GH, Corrigall VM, Panayi GS. Treatment of rheumatoid arthrits with single dose or weekly pulses of chimaeric anti-CD4 monoclonal antibody. Scand J Immunol 1992; 36:291-298.

4. Drossos AA, Lanchbury JS, Panayi GS, Moutsopoulos HM. Rheumatoid arthritis in Greek and British patients: comparative clinical,radiological, and serological study. Arthritis Rheum 1992; 35:745-748.

5. Egeland T, Lea T, Saari G, Mellbye OJ, Natvig JB. Quantitation of cells secreting rheumatoid factor of IgG, IgA and IgM class after elution from rheumatoid synovial tissue. Arthritis Rheum 1982; 25:1445-1450.

6. Elliott MJ, Maini RN, Feldmann M, et al. Treatment of rheumatoid arthritis with chimeric monoclonal antibodies to tumor necrosis factor alpha. Arthritis & Rheum 1993; 12:1681-1690.

7. Emery P, Panayi GS, Huston G, et al. D-penicillamine induced toxicity in rheumatoid arthritis: the role of sulphoxidation status and HLA-DR3. J Rheumatol 1984; 11:626-632.

8. Fischer HP, Sharrock CEM, Colston MJ, Panayi GS. Limiting dilution analysis of proliferative T cell responses to mycobacterial 65-kDa heat-shock protein fails to show significant frequency differences between synovial fluid and peripheral blood of patients with rheumatoid arthritis. Eur J Immunol 1991; 21:2937-2941.

9. Gough A, Faint J, Salmon M, et al. Genetic typing of patients with inflammatory arthritis as presentation can be used to predict outcome. Arthritis & Rheum 1994; 37:1166-1170.

10. Gregersen PK, Silver J, Winchester RJ. The shared epitope hypothesis. An approach to understanding the molecular genetics of susceptibility to rheumatoid arthritis. Arthritis Rheum 1987; 30:1205-1213.

11.   Katsikis PD, Chu Cong-Qui, Brennan FM, Maini RN, Feldmann M. Immunoregulatory
      role of interleukin 10 in rheumatoid arthritis. J exp Med 1994; 179:1517-1527.

12.   Kavanaugh AF, Davis LS, Nichols LA, et al. Treatment of refractory rheumatoid
      arthritis with a monoclonal antibody to intercellular adhesion molecule 1. Arthritis &
      Rheum 1994; 37:992-999.

13.   Keffer J, Probert L, Cazlaris H, et al. Transgenic mice expressing human tumour
      necrosis factor: a predictive genetic model of arthritis. EMBO J 1991; 10:4025-4031.

14.   Kirkham BW, Thien F, Pelton BK, et al. Chimeric CD7 monoclonal antibody therapy
      in rheumatoid arthritis. J Rheumatol 1992; 19:1348-1352.

15.   Klimiuk PS, Clague RB, Grennan DM, Dyer PA, Smeaton I, Harris R. Autoimmunity
      to native type II collagen: A distinct genetic subset of rheumatoid arthritis. J Rheumatol
      1985; 12:865-870.

16.   Koch AE, Harlow LA, Haines GK, et al. Vasular endothelial growth factor. A cytokine
      modulating endothelial function in rheumatoid arthritis. J Immunol 1994; 4149-4156.

17.   Lanchbury JSS, Jaeger EEM, Sansom DM, et al. Strong primary selection for the Dw4
      subtype of DR4 accounts for the HLA-DQw7 association with Felty's syndrome. Human
      Immunology 1991; 32:56-64.

18.   Laskin RS. Total condylar knee replacement in patients who have rheumatoid arthritis.
      A ten year follow-up study. J Bone Jt Surg (Am) 1991; 72:529-535.

19.   Moreland LW, Pratt PW, Bucy RP, Jackson BS, Feldman JW, Koopman WJ. Treatment
      of refractory rheumatoid arthritis with a chimeric anti-CD4 monoclonal antibody.
      Arthritis & Rheum 1994; 37:834-838.

20.   Panayi GS, Lanchbury JS, Kingsley GH. The importance of the T cell in inititiating and
      maintaining the chronic synovitis of rheumatoid arthritis. Arthritis Rheum 1992;
      35:729-735.

21.   Pitzalis C, Kingsley GH, Murphy J, Panayi GS. Abnormal distribution of the
      helper-inducer and suppressor-inducer T lymphocyte subsets in the rheumatoid joint. Clin
      Immunol Immunopathol 1987; 45:252-258.

22.   Poulter LW, Duke O, Hobbs S, Janossy G, Panayi GS. The involvement of
      interdigitating (antigen-presenting) cells in the pathogenesis of rheumatoid arthritis. Clin
      Exp Immunol 1983; 51:247-254.

23.   Scott DL, Panayi GS, Van Riel PLCM, Smolen J, van-de Putte-LB. Disease activity in rheumatoid arthritis: preliminary report of the Consensus Study Group of the European Workshop for Rheumatology Research. Clin Exp Rheumatol 1992; 10:521-525.

24.   Van Leeuvan MA, Van der Heijde DM, Van Rijswijk MH, et al. Interrelationship of outcome measures and process variables in early rheumatoid arthritis. J Rheumatol 1994; 21:425-429.

25.   Williams RO, Mason LJ, Feldmann M, Maini RN. Synergy between anti-CD4 and anti-tumor necrosis factor in the amelioration of established collagen-induced arthritis. Proceedings of the National Academy of Sciences of the United States of America 1994; 91:2762-2766.

AAS 47
Inflammation:
Mechanisms and Therapeutics
© 1995 Birkhäuser Verlag Basel

IMMUNOGLOBULIN GENE EXPRESSION IN RHEUMATOID ARTHRITIS

S. Louis Bridges, Jr., William J. Koopman, Soo Kon Lee, Björn E. Clausen, Perry M. Kirkham, Charles H. Rundle, and Harry W. Schroeder, Jr.

University of Alabama at Birmingham and Birmingham Veterans Administration Medical Center, Birmingham, Alabama, USA

SUMMARY: Rheumatoid arthritis (RA) is characterized by inflammation of synovium, in which immunoglobulin-secreting plasma cells are generally present. The forces driving immunoglobulin expression in RA synovium are unknown. Sequences of VH and Vκ transcripts from an RA synovial cDNA library demonstrate patterns of somatic mutation typical of an antigen-driven response. Moreover, 5% of the κ repertoire appears to derive from the same B cell progenitor, suggesting an oligoclonal response. Immunoglobulin expression in this synovium thus appears to result from antigen stimulation. In addition, this patient's synovium is enriched for unusually long Vκ-Jκ joins (CDR3s), suggesting abnormal selection or regulation of the B cell response in RA.

INTRODUCTION

Rheumatoid arthritis (RA) is a chronic inflammatory disease characterized by lymphocytic infiltration of the synovial membrane of the joints, which often leads to joint destruction (1). In longstanding RA, synovial tissue often contains germinal center-like structures similar to those seen in normal secondary lymphoid organs such as spleen (2). As many as 15% of the inflammatory cells in RA synovium are mature B lymphocytes or actively secreting plasma cells (3). Immunoglobulins secreted in synovial tissue may form immune complexes that are deposited in cartilage and contribute to tissue injury (1,4). Because the pattern of immunoglobulin gene expression reflects the forces that shape the B cell response, analysis of the synovial antibody repertoire can yield insight into the pathogenesis of the inflammatory response in RA synovium.

Immunoglobulins are heterodimeric proteins consisting of two identical heavy chains and two identical light chains (5,6). Each chain has a variable domain that recognizes antigen, and one to four constant domains that carry out effector function. In humans, antibody heavy chain gene assembly takes place in the bone marrow and procedes in a stepwise fashion. Assembly begins with DH→JH joining, followed by VH→DH-JH rearrangement, resulting in formation of a complete H chain variable domain [Reviewed in (7)].

The human VH locus on chromosome 14 is complex, containing ~90 gene segments approximately 50 of which are potentially functional (8,9). These VH gene segments can be grouped into seven families (designated VH1 through VH7), in which members share greater than 80% nucleotide sequence homology with each other. VH families range in size from multisequence families such as VH3 (about 30 members) to the single member VH6 family. There are approximately 30 DH gene segments and 6 known JH gene segments [reviewed in (7)].

Typically light chain gene rearrangement follows production of a functional H chain domain. There are two types of light chains, κ and λ. Initial rearrangements most commonly occur in the κ locus, with joining of a Vκ to a Jκ gene segment. The κ locus on chromosome 2 contains approximately 85 Vκ gene segments (35 potentially functional), 5 Jκ gene segments, and a single Cκ gene (10). Four major Vκ families have been recognized in man, ranging in size from more than 30 members (VκI) to a family with a single member (VκIV) (10,11).

Although Vλ-Jλ rearrangement can precede rearrangement in the κ locus, it most commonly occurs in pre-B cells that have failed to generate a functional κ light chain. The lambda locus is the least well characterized of the immunoglobulin loci. There are ~50 Vλ gene segments which can be grouped into at least ten families and four functional Cλ constant domains, each with its own Jλ (12).

A combination of genetic and somatic mechanisms allows the generation of a highly diverse repertoire of antigen binding sites from a limited number of germline gene segments (5). Diversity is generated in part by the ability to manufacture variable domains from random combinations of V, D, and J gene segments and the ability to combine different heavy and light chains. The insertion of non-germline encoded nucleotides at sites of rearrangement of immunoglobulin genes is another mechanism of generating diversity. The enzyme terminal deoxynucleotidyl transferase

(TdT) is responsible for this process, termed N region addition. TdT is typically detected in B lineage cells only prior to production of a functional heavy chain (13). N region addition, in association with variable degrees of exonucleolytic cleavage of nucleotides at the termini of the V, D, and J gene segments, generates heavy chain VDJ junctions that vary tremendously in length, structure and sequence (14). In the mouse, the absence of D gene segments and the lack of N region addition results in minimal Vκ-Jκ junctional diversity. The absence of N region addition has been attributed to the lack of detectable TdT protein in cells at the time of kappa light chain rearrangement. However, data from our laboratories and others have found surprisingly frequent N region addition in Vκ transcripts (15,16) suggesting that TdT may have been present in quantities below the limits of detection by serologic techniques.

Comparisons of VH and VL sequences have shown that each variable domain contains three sequence intervals of hypervariability, known as complementarity determining regions (CDRs), that are separated from each other by four regions of relatively constant sequence, termed framework regions (FRs). The V gene segment encodes CDRs 1 and 2, whereas CDR3 is the product of V-D-J joining (or V-J joining in the light chain). X-ray crystallographic solution of the crystal structure of immunoglobulins has shown that the FRs provide a structural scaffold that holds the heavy and light chain CDRs together to form the antigen binding site (6). The V-encoded CDR1 and CDR2 regions form the outside border, and the somatically generated CDR3 regions form the center of the antigen binding site. The central position of the CDR3 domains explains their essential role in defining antigen specificity. Because each CDR3 sequence results from a unique V(D)J rearrangement event that includes random N region addition, CDR3 nucleotide sequence identity defines clonal relatedness of transcripts.

Somatic hypermutation, the process of nucleotide substitutions in the germline sequences of immunoglobulin heavy and light chains, can introduce novel sequence throughout the V domain, exponentially increasing the potential diversity of the repertoire (5). Because of redundancy in the genetic code, a given mutation may give rise to a codon that encodes the same amino acid residue as the original germline sequence. This type of mutation is termed a silent (S) mutation. Alternatively, a mutation may alter the amino acid residue encoded by the germline sequence. This type of mutation is referred to as a replacement (R) mutation.

Analysis of antibody repertoires expressed in an autoimmune disease such as RA can yield insight into the mechanisms that have generated an abnormal humoral response. The two major theories proposed to explain the humoral response in autoimmune diseases have attributed autoantibody production to either polyclonal activation of bystander B cells or to antigen-driven B cell selection resulting in oligoclonal expansion. The polyclonal activation theory holds that antibodies result from activation of multiple B lymphocyte clones expressing a wide variety of specificities (17). In contrast, the antigen-driven model invokes one or more antigens as stimuli for pathogenic antibody production (18).

Studies in animal models have provided significant insight into the characteristics of antigen-driven responses (18,19). Oligoclonal expansion of antigen-specific cells results in the production of predominantly class-switched antibodies with non-random utilization of particular V gene segments. Succeeding generations of B lineage cells introduce new somatic mutations into the V domains with replacement mutations concentrated in the CDRs (the primary sites of antigen recognition). For example, antibodies of a secondary response typically have replacement to silent (R/S) mutation ratios of less than 2.9 in their FRs. In contrast, the CDRs demonstrate R/S ratios of greater than 2.9, presumably due to positive selection for somatically generated, high affinity antigen binding sites (18-20). Within a germinal center that is responding to an antigen, variable domains with shared mutations can often be found. Cells expressing these mutations are subsequently selected on the basis of increased affinity for antigen. This process of positive selection of antibodies containing novel mutations that confer enhanced antigen affinity is referred to as affinity maturation (18).

ANALYSIS OF VH GENE SEGMENT UTILIZATION IN RHEUMATOID ARTHRITIS BY *IN SITU* HYBRIDIZATION

We have used *in situ* hybridization to examine patterns of heavy chain V region gene expression in RA synovial and peripheral blood B cells (C. H. Rundle, manuscript in preparation). We generated oligonucleotide probes based on germline sequences of FR2 or FR3 of each human VH family (21). Each probe was tested by Southern hybridization to a panel of 30 germline and mutated cDNAs representing each family and by *in situ* hybridization to a panel of 17 sequenced

B cell lines representing each family. The sensitivity and specificity of each probe for its corresponding VH family was excellent. Peripheral blood lymphocytes (PBLs) from 7 normal individuals and from 7 patients with RA were stimulated *in vitro* with pokeweed mitogen (PWM) and VH gene family distribution determined by *in situ* hybridization. In addition, single cell suspensions were prepared from synovia obtained from 5 additional RA patients and compared by *in situ* hybridization to PWM-stimulated PBL from each patient. The frequency of VH gene family expression in the PBL from controls and PBLs from RA patients was similar and appeared to be the result of random utilization of VH gene families. The VH families with the most numerous germline members were more frequently expressed (VH1, 16%; VH3, 42%; VH4, 20%) than those with fewer members (VH2, 4%; VH5, 7%; VH6, 3%). The VH7 family, when present, was expressed at a frequency of approximately 3%.

Of note, the distribution of VH gene family expression in RA synovia differed from paired PBL samples. In the five patients studied, the VH7 gene family was found to predominate in 3 synovia (approximately 58% of the total VH positive cells). Members of the VH4 family were most frequently utilized in synovium from the fourth patient (40% of the total VH positive cells). In the fifth patient, from whom synovial samples of two joints were obtained simultaneously, no single VH family predominated in the synovia. However, there were higher than expected levels of expression of members of the VH1 family in both of this patient's synovia relative to his PBLs. Of interest, the VH family distributions were similar in the two synovia from this patient. The skewed distribution of VH gene family expression in the synovia is consistent with local immune responses which are antigen driven.

MOLECULAR BASIS OF ANTIBODY PRODUCTION IN RHEUMATOID ARTHRITIS SYNOVIUM

In order to examine the nature of the antibody repertoire expressed in RA synovium at the nucleotide sequence level, we generated two oligo d(T)-primed cDNA libraries from mRNA of unselected cells from synovial tissue of a 62 year old white female with longstanding active RA. It is expected that the majority of immunoglobulin transcripts were derived from plasma cells, because transcript representation in a randomly primed cDNA library reflects mRNA abundance and plasma cells express 150-1000 fold higher transcript levels per cell than their pre-B cell progenitors (22). Thus, this approach permitted us to analyze variable domain utilization, patterns of somatic mutation, and clonal relationships of immunoglobulins transcribed by activated B lineage cells in inflamed RA synovium without bias due to preferential transformation or cell growth under *in vitro* conditions.

Sequence analysis was performed on a random sample of 15 Vκ-containing recombinants (15). Nine (60%) were derived from VκI gene segments. Of the remaining six clones, all were derived from VκIII gene segments: three from Humkv328, two from Vg, and one from Humkv325. None of the other six potentially functional germline VκIII gene segments were isolated in this sample of clones. All three of the VκIII gene segments found in this library have been reported to encode rheumatoid factors. Humkv328 encodes the 6B6.6 cross-reactive idiotype (CRI) and Humkv325 encodes the 17.109 CRI, both of which are frequently associated with paraproteins expressing rheumatoid factor activity (23). The κ variable domains contained numerous somatic mutations (92-97% nucleotide sequence homology to germline). Unexpectedly, 29% of the Vκ-Jκ joins contained N region addition. The combination of N region addition and variation in the sites of Vκ-Jκ splicing led to a relatively high proportion of CDR3 regions of unusual length. CDR3 regions containing 11 amino acid codons were found in 18% of the clones.

Further screening of these libraries revealed that the kappa light chain repertoire in this patient's synovial tissue was enriched for transcripts derived from Humkv325 (24). Of 55 Cκ+ clones analyzed, 8 (15%) were derived from this gene segment (Fig. 1). These sequences contained high R/S ratios in the CDRs compared to FRs. The R/S ratios for all Humkv325-derived clones were: CDR1, 3.0; CDR2, 8.0; CDR3, 1.4; FR1, 0.3; FR2, 0.7; FR3, 1.1; FR4, 0.5. These changes suggest an antigen-driven response. More definitive evidence of an oligoclonal response came from identification of a set of three κ light chains with identical coding sequence throughout the entire Vκ and Jκ regions (Fig. 1). In these cDNA libraries from the synovial tissue of a patient with longstanding RA, 3 of 64 (5%) of the Cκ[+] sequences were apparently derived from the same progenitor B cell (24).

A.

```
           |<--                              CDR3                    -->|  FR4->
Codon       89   90   91   92   93   94   95      95A  95B     96   97
Humkv325   CAG  CAG  TAT  GGT  AGC  TCA  CCT  CC|<--N-->|<-- Jκ    -->
 *10S2     ...  ..C  ...  ...  G..  ,.G  ...  .      GG   GA   . ... ...
 *21S2     ...  ..C  ...  ...  G..  ..G  ...  .      GG   GA   . ... ...
 *38S1     ...  ..C  ...  ...  G..  ..G  ...  .      GG   GA   . ... ...
  28S1     ...  ...  ...  ...  GA.  ...  ...  .                .. ...
  37S4     ...  ...  ...  ...  GA.  ..C  ..         A    A     .. ...
  25S5     ..T  .G.  ...  ..A  .C.  ...  ...  ..              . ... ...
  25S4     ...  ...  ...  ...  ..T  ...  T.G                  ... ...
  16S1     ..C  ...  ...  ..A  TAT  A..  ..C  .               .. ...
```

B.

```
           |<--          CDR3              -->|<-- FR4  -->|
Codon       89              95A  95B      96   98         107
Humkv325   QQYGSSP                        |<--  Jκ    -->|
 *10S2     .H..G..          R    E         ..  .......... Jκ2
 *21S2     .H..G..          R    E         ..  .......... Jκ2
 *38S1     .H..G..          R    E         ..  .......... Jκ2
  28S1     ....D..                         R.  .......... Jκ1
  37S4     ....D..          R               .  .......... Jκ1
  25S5     HR..T..          P              ..  .......... Jκ5
  25S4     ......S                         ..  .........R Jκ2
  16S1     H...YT.                         ..  ..A....... Jκ4
```

Figure 1. A. Nucleotide sequences of CDR3 regions of eight Humkv325 derived clones are compared to the germline Humkv325 sequence or the corresponding Jκ gene segment. Dots denote germline identity. Nucleotides at the Vκ-Jκ junctions that could not be assigned to either the Vκ or Jκ gene segments are identified as the likely products of N region addition. B. The deduced amino acid sequences are represented in single letter code, with a dot denoting identity to the germline Humkv325 sequence or to corresponding Jκ. * The CDR3 regions of clones 10S2, 21S2 and 38S1 are identical to each other and as a result of N region addition are 11 amino acids in length. Adapted from Reference (24).

To analyze the heavy chain repertoire in these libraries from a single individual with RA, we initially performed Southern blot analysis for VH and JH utilization on the first 50 $C\gamma^+$ and JH^+ recombinants and selected a set of clones at random for sequence analysis (25). The majority of transcripts from this synovial sample contained gene segments derived from the larger VH families: VH1 (28%), VH3 (56%), and VH4 (15%). However, sequencing of additional clones has identified one transcript from the VH2 family, one from the VH5 family, and one from the VH6 family. These results are in general agreement with our *in situ* hybridization studies discussed above. There was a predominance of JH4, JH5, and JH6 gene segment utilization among transcripts from these two cDNA libraries. Eight of 14 (57%) VH gene segments were most closely related to those that are preferentially expressed in human fetal liver or that encode antibodies with self-reactivity. The V domains were heavily mutated, with high R/S ratios in the CDRs. CDR3 lengths were quite variable, due to extensive N region addition and 5' exonuclease activity in the VH-DH-JH joins. More in-depth sequence analysis revealed that three of 68 Cγ^+ clones were identical to each other suggesting that, as in the κ light chain repertoire, approximately 5% of the heavy chains are derived from the same progenitor B cell (B. E. Clausen et al, manuscript in preparation).

We next sought to determine if the clonally expanded κ light chains isolated from this patient's synovium were also expressed in her peripheral blood lymphocytes or in normal controls. Using the polymerase chain reaction (PCR), we amplified Vκ transcripts from cDNA of the patient's synovial tissue, her PBLs obtained within 24 hours of joint replacement, from PBLs of a normal 32 year old white male, and from cadaveric spleen cells of a 49 year old white male without rheumatic disease. We enriched the PCR products for Humkv325-derived transcripts by using a 5' primer based on the germline leader and FR1 of Humkv325. PCR products from each of these samples were probed with oligonucleotide probes specific for the CDR3 region of the clonally expanded κ light chain (24). κ light chains containing this CDR3 region were detected only in the patient's synovial tissue. These findings suggest that the expansion of B cells in this autoimmune disease is likely the product of local antigen-driven selection.

Vκ DOMAINS EXPRESSED IN RHEUMATOID ARTHRITIS ARE ENRICHED FOR UNUSUALLY LONG CDR3 REGIONS

To determine if increased amounts of N region addition and unusually long CDR3 regions are associated with RA, we subcloned and sequenced Vκ domains from the PCR reactions described above. In addition, we studied Vκ domains expressed in PBLs of a normal 60 year old white female to serve as an age, sex, and race-matched control for our initial RA patient. Of a total of 62 Vκ-containing clones from these tissues, 90% were derived from VκIII gene segments.

Transcripts from RA synovium and PBLs contained more N region addition than those from controls. The percentages of clones with at least one base pair of N region addition were surprisingly high: 62 WF RA Synovium 7 of 14 (50%), 62 WF RA PBL 10 of 15 (67%), 32 WM Normal PBL 5 of 12 (42%), 49 WM Spleen 5 of 10 (50%), and 60 WF Normal PBL 3 of 11 (27%).

Despite the finding of relatively frequent N region addition in the Vκ-Jκ joins of both normal individuals and those with RA, unusually long CDR3 regions were expressed only in RA-derived tissues. CDR3 regions 11 codons in length were found in 5 of 29 (17%) Vκ clones derived from synovium and PBLs of the patient with RA; none of the 33 Vκ transcripts from control tissues contained such long CDR3 regions. This finding is in stark contrast to sequences reported in the compilation by Kabat, in which none of the 56 reported human VκIII sequences (amino acid and nucleotide submissions combined) contain 11 codons (6). Preliminary analyses of 38 additional clones from additional individuals (two with RA and one normal control) have corroborated our findings of enrichment for unusually long Vκ CDR3 regions in RA (S. L. Bridges, Jr., et al, manuscript in preparation).

STRUCTURAL SIGNIFICANCE OF κ LIGHT CHAINS WITH 11 AMINO ACID CDR3 REGIONS

Introduction of additional amino acid residues into κ light chain CDR3 regions could have important ramifications with regard to antigen specificity of the antibody. To analyze possible structural changes induced by the unusually long CDR3 region, we modeled the clonally expanded kappa light chain as previously described (24). Amino acid 96, the arginine residue introduced by N region addition, was not solvent-exposed, but was buried beneath the surface of the antigen binding site. The four most closely juxtaposed amino acid residues were found to be heavy chain residues 99 and 105 (VH CDR3), light chain residue 99 (Vκ CDR3), and light chain residue 37 (Vκ FR2). Residue 96 in the CDR3 region may thus affect the conformation of the antibody binding site in one of three ways: directly, indirectly through contacts with the CDR3 of the light and heavy chain, or by internal interactions with the Vκ FR2. In addition, introduction of a charged residue at this position may influence heavy and light chain pairing.

SUMMARY

Our studies of VH and Vκ repertoires expressed in RA synovial tissue have provided support for the hypothesis that the B cell response in RA synovium is at least in part antigen-driven. We have shown by molecular analysis that there is a component of oligoclonal B cell expansion at the site of inflammation in this chronic disease. We found three identical heavy chain transcripts and three identical kappa light chain transcripts, but did not isolate any non-identical Vκ or VH sequences with shared mutations. Because of the absence of such transcripts and the longstanding nature of the inflammation in the joint of this patient, we speculate that the clonally expanded sequences represent the products of a highly focused immune response for a particular antigen.

Human κ light chain rearrangements, in contrast to those in rodents, often contain N region addition that contributes extensively to the diversity generated at sites of V→J joining. We have found that normal controls and RA patients contain a similar percentage of transcripts with N region addition at the V→J join. Despite the frequent presence of N region addition, the length of the vast majority of CDR3 regions from individuals without RA are relatively constant, with greater than 95% of κ transcripts from unselected tissues containing either 9 or 10 amino acids codons. Although CDR3 domains of 11 amino acids can be found, they appear to be rare. However, in the majority of the RA patients examined, the consequences of N region addition appear to be quite different. Vκ transcripts containing 11 amino acids in their CDR3s are more commonly found in patients with RA than in normal controls.

The enrichment for unusually long Vκ CDR3 findings may reflect abnormal development of the pre-immune repertoire in the bone marrow of RA patients, perhaps through abnormal regulation of TdT. An alternative explanation is antigen selection and clonal outgrowth of rare B cells that express antibodies bearing these unusually long Vκ CDR3 regions. In either case, it is apparent that the antibody repertoires of some RA patients are different from those of normal individuals. Expression of these abnormal antibody repertoires may play a role in the pathogenesis of RA.

ACKNOWLEDGEMENTS

The authors gratefully acknowledge the technical assistance of John Lavelle, Priscilla Fowler, and Jennifer Collins. This work was supported, in part, by a VA Merit Award (WJK) and NIH grants AR01867 (SLB), AI07051 (PMK), AR03555 (HWS and WJK), AI18958 (WJK), AI18745 (WJK), AR20614 (WJK), DK40117 (WJK), AI23694 (HWS), AI30879 (HWS), and AI34568 (HWS).

REFERENCES

1. Zvaifler NJ. Immunopathology of joint inflammation in rheumatoid arthritis. Adv Immunol 1973; 16:265-336.

2. Ziff M. Relation of cellular infiltration of rheumatoid synovial membrane to its immune response. Arthritis Rheum 1974; 17:313-319.

3. Kobayashi I, Ziff M. Electron microscopic studies of lymphoid cells in the rheumatoid synovial membrane. Arthritis Rheum 1973; 16:471-486.

4. Harris ED, Jr. Rheumatoid arthritis: Pathophysiology and implications for therapy. New Engl J Med 1990; 322:1277-1289.

5. Tonegawa S. Somatic generation of antibody diversity. Nature. 1983; 302:575-581.

6. Kabat EA, Wu TT, Perry HM, Gottesman KS, Foeller C. Sequences of proteins of immunological interest. 5th edition. Bethesda, Maryland: U.S. Department of Health and Human Services; 1991: 1-2387.

7. Schroeder HW, Jr., Perlmutter RM. Development of the human antibody repertoire. In: New Concepts in Immunodeficiency Diseases. Gupta S, Griscelli C, editors. Chichester: John Wiley & Sons, 1993: 1-20.

8. Matsuda F, Shin EK, Nagaoka H, Matsumura R, Haino M, Fukita Y, Taka-ishi S, Imai T, Riley JH, Anand R, Soeda E, Honjo T. Structure and physical map of 64 variable segments in

the 3' 0.8-megabase region of the human immunoglobulin heavy-chain locus. Nature Genet 1993; 3:88-94.

9. Cook GP, Tomlinson IM, Walter G, Reithman H, Carter NP, Bulewela L, Winter G, Rabbitts TH. A map of the human immunoglobulin VH locus completed by analysis of the telomeric region of chromosome 14q. Nature Genet 1994; 7:162-168.

10. Meindl A, Klobeck H-G, Ohnheiser R, Zachau HG. The Vκ gene repertoire in the human germline. Eur J Immunol 1990; 20:1855-1863.

11. Klobeck H-G, Bornkamm GW, Combriato G, Mockikat R, Polenz H-D, Zachau HG. Subgroup IV of human immunoglobulin κ light chains is encoded by a single germline gene. Nucleic Acids Res 1985; 13 6515-6529.

12. Selsing E, Durdik J, Moore MW, Persiani DM. Immunoglobulin lambda genes. In: Immunoglobulin Genes. Honjo T, Alt FW, Rabbitts TH, editors. London: Academic Press, 1989: 111-122.

13. Desiderio SV, Yancopoulos GD, Paskind M, Thomas E, Boss MA, Landau N, Alt FW, Baltimore D. Insertion of N regions into heavy-chain genes is correlated with expression of terminal deoxytransferase in B cells. Nature 1984; 311:752-755.

14. Sanz I. Multiple mechanisms participate in the generation of diversity of human H chain CDR3 regions. J Immunol 1991; 147:1720-1729.

15. Lee SK, Bridges SL, Jr., Koopman WJ, Schroeder HW, Jr. The immunoglobulin kappa light chain repertoire expressed in the synovium of a patient with rheumatoid arthitis. Arthritis Rheum 1992; 35:905-913.

16. Victor KD, Capra JD. An apparently common mechanism of generating antibody diversity: length variation of the VL-JL junction. Molecular Immunology 1994; 31:39-46.

17. Hang L, Slack JH, Amundson C, Izui S, Theofilopoulos AN, Dixon FJ. Induction of murine autoimmune disease by chronic polyclonal B cell activation. J Exp Med 1983; 157:874-883.

18. Shlomchik MJ, Marshak-Rothstein A, Wolfowicz CB, Rothstein TL, Weigert MG. The role of clonal selection and somatic mutation in autoimmunity. Nature 1987; 328:805-811.

19. Shlomchik MJ, Aucoin AH, Pisetsky DS, Weigert MG. Structure and function of anti-DNA autoantibodies derived from a single autoimmune mouse. Proc Natl Acad Sci USA 1987; 84:9150-9154.

20. Shlomchik MJ, Nemazee DA, Sato VL, van Snick J, Carson DA, Weigert MG. Variable region sequences of murine IgM anti-IgG monoclonal autoantibodies (rheumatoid factors). A

structural explanation for the high frequency of IgM anti-IgG B cells. J Exp Med 1986; 164:407-427.

21. Rundle CH, Schroeder HW, Jr., Koopman WJ. Analysis of immunoglobulin VH gene family expression in rheumatoid arthritis. Arthritis Rheum 1994; 37(Suppl):S395.

22. Kelley DE, Perry RP. Transcriptional and posttranscriptional control of immunoglobulin mRNA production during B lymphocyte development. Nucleic Acids Res 1986; 14:5431-5447.

23. Crowley JJ, Goldfien RD, Schrohenloher RE, Spiegelberg HL, Silverman GJ, Mageed RA, Jefferis R, Koopman WJ, Carson DA, Fong S. Incidence of three cross-reactive idiotypes on human rheumatoid factor paraproteins. J Immunol 1988; 140:3411-3418.

24. Lee SK, Bridges SL, Jr., Kirkham PM, Koopman WJ, Schroeder HW, Jr. Evidence of antigen receptor-influenced oligoclonal B lymphocyte expansion in the synovium of a patient with longstanding rheumatoid arthritis. J Clin Invest 1994; 93:361-370.

25. Bridges SL, Jr., Lee SK, Koopman WJ, Schroeder HW, Jr. Analysis of immunoglobulin gamma heavy chain expression in synovial tissue of a patient with rheumatoid arthritis. Arthritis Rheum 1993; 36:631-641.

AAS 47
Inflammation:
Mechanisms and Therapeutics
© 1995 Birkhäuser Verlag Basel

CYTOKINE NETWORKS IN RHEUMATOID ARTHRITIS: IMPLICATIONS FOR THERAPY

Gary S. Firestein

Gensia, Inc., 9360 Towne Centre Drive, San Diego, CA 92121

I. INTRODUCTION AND HISTORICAL PERSPECTIVE

The immune system was implicated in rheumatoid arthritis (RA) fifty years ago when rheumatoid factors were first characterized as autoantibodies. For many decades after this seminal observation, synovitis research focused on the humoral aspects of immunity. More recently, the primacy of antibody responses in RA was supplanted by more sophisticated paradigms that also implicated T cells and cell mediated immunity. While the target for a putative antigen specific response was not defined, it was assumed to be either a xenoantigen (like a virus, retrovirus, or bacterial cell wall) or a self-protein. This antigen driven model of rheumatoid synovitis was supported by a host of observations, including the prevalence of helper T cells in inflamed synovium and, perhaps more compelling, exquisitely defined associations with specific major histocompatibility proteins. The latter data certainly steer one towards the nearly inescapable conclusion that such associations are defined by the topography of the antigen-binding groove of HLA-DR and the structure of a putative "rheumatoid antigen."

These models have served workers in the field for quite some time and led to an explosion of information regarding the properties and actions of synovial tissue and synovial fluid T cells. However, the utility of a model should also be judged by its ability to direct one towards successful therapeutic interventions. Despite widely disseminated proclamations to the contrary, novel therapies that draw on this paradigm have enjoyed only a modicum of success. Many "T cell-specific" therapies have actually been a disappointment in the clinic. For instance, anti-T cell antibodies (including anti-CD4, anti-CD5, anti-CAMPATH, and others) have not provided the expected benefit; nor have total nodal irradiation, thoracic drug drainage, or even agents like cyclosporin that are such potent immunosuppressive agents that they can prevent allograft rejection.

In the mid-1980's, our understanding of the complex rheumatoid process advanced with the advent of cytokine biology. In its infancy, the study of cytokines in rheumatoid arthritis suggested that T cells generated a plethora of lymphokines that drove synovitis. However, early cytokine studies in RA were flawed by reliance on biological assays; later studies showed that T cell products were actually present only in very low concentrations (see below). In contrast, factors produced by other cell types, especially macrophages and fibroblasts, were abundant. This has led to new paradigms for RA that attempt to incorporate these observations.

II. CYTOKINES AND RA: TECHNICAL ISSUES OF ASSAY DEVELOPMENT

Cytokines are hormone-like proteins that enable immune cells to communicate with one another. In the early days of cytokine biology, assays relied on biological responses, such as proliferation of cytokine-dependent cell lines. What was not appreciated at the time was the general lack of specificity of these assays. For instance, some IL-2-dependent cell lines were later discovered to respond to IL-4, and IL-1-dependent cells were also stimulated by IL-6 and other cytokines. This problem was greatly compounded by the use of complex biological samples like synovial fluid that contain a mixture of factors. Such artifacts probably account for the early discovery of gamma-interferon-like activity in synovial fluid, which was likely due to the action of other factors (especially IL-6) now known to be present in very high concentrations. The use of bioassays in combination with newer reagents, like monoclonal antibodies that neutralize specific cytokines or their receptors, helped clarify some of these issues (1). However, other problems, including the presence of soluble receptors or even natural anti-cytokine antibodies, only added to the difficulty interpreting bioassays of synovial fluid.

In the late 1980's, the first immunoassays were used to study cytokine levels in synovial fluid (2). Although occasionally less sensitive than bioassays, specificity was greatly enhanced. Some problems were not entirely overcome by this technology. For instance, soluble receptors can potentially interfere with antibody binding and the concentrations of certain membrane bound cytokines might be underestimated. Additional problems that are specific to measuring cytokines in rheumatoid synovial fluids have been encountered. The high viscosity of synovial fluid impairs sensitivity of solid phase ELISAs by limiting diffusion of cytokines to the antibody-coated surfaces; this can be ameliorated by pre-treating fluids with enzymes like hyaluronidase. Proteases in synovial fluid can also interfere with cytokine detection if they modify antigenic sites on the target protein. The presence of rheumatoid factors is an even more daunting obstacle. Rheumatoid factors can potentially cross link the Fc portions of antibodies used in immunoassays (especially when rabbit antibodies are used) and can cause false positive readings. The extent of this complication should not be underestimated and its occurrence does not correlate with the presence of rheumatoid factor in peripheral blood. Even with these problems, however, immunoassays are now the gold standard for detecting cytokines in biological samples.

Other methods of detection that have become increasingly prevalent involve the use of molecular biology to detect specific cytokine RNA transcripts. While cumbersome and time consuming, these methods provide a level of specificity that has previously eluded the field. A measure of caution is required here, too, since mRNA accumulation does not always correlate with protein production. The use of reverse transcriptase-polymerase chain reaction (RT-PCR) has now enhanced the sensitivity of molecular biology techniques to the point where its utility can be questioned. Even a single copy of mRNA can be detected in some samples. While RT-PCR can potentially provide a "yes or no" answer about the presence of a particular cytokine mRNA, an errant copy of mRNA from contaminating blood cells might inadvertently be detected. Moreover, attempts to quantify cytokine mRNA by RT-PCR raise a myriad of additional issues and artifacts.

III. CYTOKINE PROFILES IN RA

Early studies of rheumatoid cytokine production focused on gamma interferon (IFN-γ). This was due, in large part, to the observation of massive amounts of HLA-DR on synovial cells. Since IFN-γ was the only known DR-inducing agent at the time, it was only natural to assume that IFN was the responsible cytokine. Viral cytopathic inhibition assays, which take advantage of the fact that the interferons (alpha, beta, and gamma) protect cells from viral infections, demonstrated IFN-like activity in synovial fluid. Surprisingly, when studies were later repeated using sensitive and specific immunoassays, only very low concentrations of IFN-γ were detected (2). Synovial fluid levels of the lymphokine were far below the amounts needed to induce HLA-DR expression on monocytes. Furthermore, neutralizing antibodies to IFN-γ did not block the ability of synovial fluid to induce HLA-DR expression on cultured monocytes. The relative lack of IFN-γ in rheumatoid joints has since been confirmed (3), including studies employing RT-PCR to detect specific RNA transcripts. The difficulty detecting IFN-γ in RA does not appear to be due to methodological problems since it is easily measured in other diseases known to be mediated by T cells, such as tuberculous pleuritis. IFN-γ mRNA was detected in tuberculous pleura by in situ hybridization (4) but RA synovial tissue was negative using similar techniques.

Other T cell products (sometimes called "lymphokines") are also conspicuously absent from RA joint samples (see Table 1). The situation with IL-2 was similar to IFN-γ in that early studies suggested high levels of biologically active cytokine in synovial fluid using IL-2-dependent cell lines. However, when biological assays were used in conjunction with monoclonal antibodies against the IL-2 receptor, it was clear that non-IL-2 factors were responsible for this activity (1). More recently, immunoassays have also failed to detect significant amounts of IL-2 in synovial fluid (3). The same is true for virtually every other T cell-specific cytokine that has been studied in detail, including IL-3, IL-4, and TNF-β. In each case, minimal amounts of cytokine have been detected in synovial fluid or synovial tissues.

Table 1. Cytokine profile of RA

	T cell derived	Macrophage/fibroblast derived
IL-1		+
IL-2	-	
IL-3	-	
IL-4	-	
IL-6		+
IL-8		+
IL-10		+
TNF-α	-	+
TNF-β	-	
IFN-γ	-	
GM-CSF		+
G-CSF		+
M-CSF		+
TGF-β		+
IL-1ra		+

-=cytokine absent or present in very low concentration; +=cytokine readily detected

In contrast to T cells, products of macrophage-like and fibroblast-like cells are ubiquitous in RA. Virtually every mediator produced by these cells for which an assay exists has been detected in the joint, including metalloproteinases, serine proteases, cysteine proteases, complement proteins, and arachidonic acid metabolites. Whereas T cell cytokines are difficult to find, macrophage- and fibroblast-derived cytokines are abundant (5). IL-1, TNF-α, IL-6, GM-CSF, M-CSF, TGF-β, a host of chemokines (a family of cytokines with chemoattractant activities), and even macrophage-derived cytokine inhibitors like IL-10 and IL-1ra are present in RA synovial fluid and synovial tissue. In situ hybridization and immunohistochemical studies on synovial tissue have confirmed these data. Using these methods, IL-1 was detected primarily in synovial macrophages. The cellular sources of GM-CSF, TNF-α and IL-6 were more interesting, since they can be produced by activated T cells under some conditions. However, in each case, the vast majority was derived from the non-T cell population, especially macrophages (6).

IV. WHERE HAVE ALL THE LYMPHOKINES GONE?

Why are T cell products so difficult to find in rheumatoid arthritis? Surely, among the plethora of macrophage cytokines in the joint, some should have sufficient T cell-activating properties to stimulate lymphokine production! There are a variety of potential explanations for this paradox, but each remains speculative. One possibility is that the local production of suppressive factors and cytokine inhibitors overwhelms the activating effects of macrophage/fibroblast cytokines in chronic arthritis. For instance, TGF-β is known to be a potent inhibitor of T cell proliferation and appears to contribute to impaired proliferative responses by synovial fluid T cells (7). IL-1ra (a naturally occurring IL-1 antagonist) is also present in synovial fluid at concentrations sufficient to block IL-1 biological activity. IL-10, which can suppress cytokine production, is also readily demonstrated in rheumatoid synovium (8). Furthermore, soluble cytokine receptors are also found in excess in synovial fluid, sometimes at concentrations several logs greater than the native cytokine. This is particularly well documented for soluble TNF receptors and accounts for the absence of TNF-α biological activity in synovial fluid despite the presence of immunoreactive protein (3).

A second explanation for the relative lack of T cell cytokines is that the cells have entered a state of arrested activation or reached a dormant "post-activation" state. In this scenario, articular T cells could be activated by a specific stimulus (the "rheumatoid antigen"?), progress through a phase of local proliferation and cytokine release, followed by a quiescent stage resembling anergy. This notion is supported by the observation that some synovial T cells contain IL-2 mRNA even though they do not secret the protein. This phenotype (i.e., high IL-2 mRNA/low IL-2 production) is characteristic of anergic T cells.

A third explanation for the dearth of lymphokines is that synovial T cells have not encountered their specific antigen. This is almost certainly true for the vast majority of T cells in the joint. While early paradigms for RA suggested that the articular accumulation of T cells was due in large part to in situ proliferation, this notion is clearly at odds with our current understanding of adhesion molecules and cellular trafficking. Factors elaborated during rheumatoid inflammation are known to induce adhesion molecule expression on synovial endothelial cells; this results in tissue accumulation of T cells in an antigen-independent manner without local proliferation. The phenotype of synovial T cells is consistent with this model since they are enriched for mature memory helper cells (the CD4 positive, CD45RO positive subset). Hence, the movement of lymphocytes from the circulation into the joint is not a random process. Adhesion molecules like ICAM-1 and VCAM-1 are expressed in great abundance in synovium. The ligands for ICAM-1 and VCAM-1 (the β2 integrins and α4/β1 integrin, respectively) are expressed on all T cells, but in significantly greater amounts on mature memory cells. Cells with this phenotype would tend to enter the inflamed synovium regardless of antigen specificity. The large number of adhesion molecules found in the synovial matrix and expressed on the surface of resident synoviocytes would favor retention of cells. Therefore, antigen-independent forces are involved in sequestering T cells in the synovium. There is little evidence of subsequent T cell proliferation within the joint; those few cells that actively synthesize DNA are enriched for the CD8 subpopulation rather than CD4 cells.

What about the minority of antigen-specific T cells that potentially orchestrate the inflammatory response? Based on animal and human studies, antigen specific cells in an immune response comprise only a small percentage of the total number of T cells, perhaps less than 1% of lymphocytes at an inflamed site. These cells might release cytokines into the microenvironment in amounts below the sensitivity of currently available assays. Alternatively, cytokines might not be released by these activated cells but remain bound to cell membranes. Given the observations of abundant T cell-derived IL-2, IFN-γ, and GM-CSF in other inflammatory diseases like tuberculosis and asthma, these explanations are more difficult to support, albeit certainly possible.

One final consideration is that the T cells do not produce cytokines in RA because chronic rheumatoid arthritis is independent of T cells. This seemingly heretical paradigm suggests that the process can be perpetuated by either transformed cells that proliferate autonomously or by the cytokine network itself. Indeed, there is some evidence that rheumatoid synoviocytes exhibit some characteristics of transformed cells, including anchorage-independent growth. Also, the cytokines known to be present in the actively inflamed joint have the potential for establishing a self-perpetuating process or contributing to autonomous cell proliferation.

V. UPDATING THE PARADIGM: THE ROLE OF NON-T CELLS

To accommodate new information on the cytokine profile into current concepts of rheumatoid arthritis, a variety of alternative models have been proposed. A central theme of these paradigms is that the chronic inflammatory process achieves a certain degree of autonomy that permits inflammation to persist after a T cell response has ended or at least been relegated to a lesser role. This hypothesis suggests that inflammation can be sustained by factors produced by neighboring macrophages and synovial fibroblasts in the joint lining in paracrine or autocrine networks. Several cytokines that have been identified in the synovium or synovial fluid can participate in this system and might explain lining cell hyperplasia, HLA-DR induction, and synovial angiogenesis. While the litany of potential actors in this drama is extensive, most would agree that IL-1 and TNFα play lead roles. Both are produced by synovial macrophages and stimulate synovial fibroblast proliferation and secretion of IL-6, GM-CSF, chemokines (like IL-8) and a panoply of effector molecules (like metalloproteinases and prostaglandins). GM-CSF, which is produced by both synovial macrophages and IL-1β- or TNF-α-stimulated synovial fibroblasts, can in turn induce IL-1 secretion to form a positive feedback loop. This is only a representative example of a complex process that involves many other cytokines. GM-CSF also increases HLA-DR expression on macrophages, perhaps explaining the high expression of this molecule in the absence of IFN-γ. TNF-α synergizes with GM-CSF as an inducer of HLA-DR on macrophages, and might contribute to macrophage class II MHC expression. Macrophage and fibroblast cytokines could also indirectly contribute to local T cell and B cell activation.

It is important to recognize that this model for the perpetuation of RA does not eliminate the possibility that synovitis is initiated by an antigen driven process. In fact, unless arthritis is truly caused by transformed cells, it requires an external stimulus to initiate (and perhaps intermittently re-stimulate) the entire process. T cell mediated responses, either directed against an inciting antigen or a secondary target (like type II collagen or proteoglycans) can occur in parallel with the macrophage/fibroblast axis and might contribute to the inflammatory milieu. While the language spoken by macrophages and fibroblasts in this dialogue is reasonably well understood, the lexicon of synovial T cells remains unknown. One additional prediction of this updated model is that the role of T cells and antigen specific processes might vary depending on the phase of the disease. For instance, early RA (i.e., the first few weeks or months of disease) might be highly dependent on T cell proliferation or activation. When the disease progresses, antigen independent processes might become more important as cytokine networks become established. What is not known, however, is how (or if) T cells interact with their neighbors in chronic disease.

VI. THERAPEUTIC IMPLICATIONS OF CYTOKINE NETWORKS

The rather unimpressive clinical results of "anti-T cell" therapy, in combination with recent data on the cytokine profile in RA, implies that alternative treatment strategies should be considered based on the revised paradigm. New approaches that interfere with cytokines can be divided into several different categories, each of which offers potential for interrupting rheumatoid synovitis. Given current knowledge of cytokines in RA, the focus today should probably be on macrophage or fibroblast derived products. The trick is to identify the pivotal cytokine (or cytokines) and use a technology that will permit modulation but not interfere with normal immune responses. Potential approaches for modifying the cytokine network are delineated below (see Table 2).

Table 2.   Therapeutic strategies aimed at cytokines

---

    1.   Inhibit cytokine production
           a. Transcription
           b. Translation
           c. Post-translational processing
    2.   Inhibit cytokine action
           a. Neutralize cytokines
           b. Interfere with receptor interactions
    3.   Inhibit signal transduction
    4.   Administer suppressive cytokines
    5.   Block consequences of cytokines
           a. Proteases
           b. Adhesion molecules
           c. Small molecule mediators (e.g., prostaglandins)

A. Inhibit cytokine production

Modulation of cytokine production in vivo is a worthy goal, albeit difficult to achieve. For instance, specific molecules can be designed to block transcription of individual cytokine genes, as with anti-sense oligonucleotides. Inadequate cell penetration and a short blood half life have limited the application of anti-sense technology in chronic systemic diseases. More traditional medicinal chemistry has met with greater success, and compounds that interfere with cytokine transcription have shown promise. Heterocyclic compounds that inhibit TNF-α (but not IL-1 or IL-6) gene expression are examples of this approach. One of these compounds has already been used successfully in a model of murine endotoxic shock (9). Tenidap is another molecule that exhibits a direct action on cytokine production in addition to its anti-inflammatory effects through inhibition of cyclo-oxygenase. The mechanism of cytokine inhibition appears to be due to interference with anion transport in activated cells. In clinical studies, tenidap also decreases synovial metalloproteinase gene expression, perhaps due to lower levels of IL-1 and TNF-α in the joint. Other sophisticated methods of inhibiting cytokine transcription are also being studied, including targeting specific gene promoters or nuclear transcription factors. Cytokine production can also be down regulated by inhibiting post-translational processing since some cytokines are produced as pro-factors that require proteolytic cleavage for activation. IL-1β is one example since it is synthesized as an inactive protein that must be modified by the enzyme IL-1 convertase. Assuming that IL-1ß is more important than IL-1α (which is biologically active even before processing), small molecule inhibitors of this enzyme could have therapeutic utility in RA. A similar approach to TNF processing enzymes might also be useful.

B. Inhibit cytokine action

1. Neutralizing cytokines

After cytokines have been produced, one might absorb or neutralize them, thereby interrupting the cytokine network. Monoclonal antibodies represent a method of neutralizing critical cytokines using readily available technology. One potential problem is the subsequent production of endogenous antibodies that neutralize the anti-cytokine antibody, thereby negating the beneficial effects over time. Also, one should consider the possibility that antibodies might actually deliver cytokines to cells rather than simply neutralize them. Since some actions of cytokines, such as TNF-α, can be mediated by direct intracellular micro-injection, the intracellular delivery of cytokines could have unexpected results. Nevertheless, encouraging results in pre-clinical animal models using anti-TNF antibodies suggest that this approach to RA might be viable (10). In addition, early clinical data in RA patients support a role for anti-TNF antibody therapy (11). An alternative approach to antibodies is to use soluble cytokine receptors or receptor/Fc fusion proteins to absorb or neutralize cytokines. This is also the subject of intense investigation using engineered IL-1 and TNF-α receptors.

2. Inhibit cytokine binding to receptor

Cytokines mediate many of their actions through interactions with high affinity surface receptors. Hence, interfering with ligand:receptor binding represents another potential therapeutic approach. This could be accomplished either with small molecules or naturally occurring inhibitors. The former has been difficult to achieve for a variety of reasons, not the least of which is the size and complexity of cytokine/receptor binding sites. A promising approach resulted from the discovery of a naturally occurring IL-1 antagonist. The IL-1 receptor antagonist (IL-1ra), competitively inhibits IL-1α and IL-1β binding to IL-1 receptors (IL-1R) (12,13). IL-1ra is a pure receptor antagonist since it does not induce signal transduction or internalization of the ligand-receptor complex. Intracellular and secreted forms of IL-1ra have been identified that result from alternative splicing of mRNA. Although IL-1ra binds to the IL-1R with high affinity, 10- to 100-fold excess IL-1ra is needed to inhibit IL-1 biological action because target cells respond when only a small percentage of IL-1R is occupied by IL-1. A controlled trial of IL-1ra in RA is underway, although the very high levels of IL-1ra needed to block the IL-1 biological response suggests that success will be difficult to achieve.

3. Inhibit signal transduction

As noted above, many cytokine actions are mediated through specific cell surface receptors. Subsequent to binding, a signal is sent to the interior of the cell through a variety of second messengers. A full discussion of these intracellular signaling mechanisms is beyond the scope of this review, although protein kinases, GTPase coupled proteins, NO synthase, and adenylate cyclase represent a few of the potential targets. Many of these targets are amenable to standard medicinal chemistry. Specificity will be a major issue if one is to avoid toxicity since many cytokines, soluble mediators, and other intracellular processes use these proteins to regulate diverse cell functions.

4. Inhibitory cytokines

Positive feedback loops in cytokine networks are balanced by suppressive factors that normally down regulate the immune response. This helps maintain homeostasis and represents a potential target for novel treatment modalities. Surprisingly, IFN-γ is one of the best characterized participants in negative feedback loops. Originally thought to be a pivotal pro-inflammatory factor in RA, IFN-γ is actually a potent inhibitor of cytokine-mediated synoviocyte activation, especially by TNF-α (14). The relative lack of IFN-γ in the rheumatoid synovium might result in unopposed TNF-α stimulation and paradoxically contribute to the disease perpetuation. IFN-γ has been tested in controlled trials in RA and demonstrates modest clinical benefit (albeit probably no more effective than "anti-T cell" therapies) (15). This is strikingly different from multiple sclerosis, where IFN-γ increases the frequency and severity of disease flares (16).

Other inhibitory cytokines could also be used to treat RA by virtue of their anti-inflammatory effects. A legitimate case could be made for treating patients with IL-4 since this cytokine inhibits synovial cytokine and protease production in vitro. Like IFN-γ, IL-4 is a T cell product that appears to be deficient in the joint and whose absence might contribute to synovitis. TGF-β also has potential due to its immunosuppressive actions, but it is a complex factor whose effects depend greatly on the concentrations used and the mode of administration. In various animal models of arthritis, TGF-β can either exacerbate or ameliorate the disease. Hence, decisions on therapeutic trials with TGF-β are fraught with potential problems. In addition, very large amounts of TGF-β are already present in the articular cavity, which raises some questions regarding the benefit of administering additional amounts of the growth factor. IL-10 also has potent anti-cytokine activity and could be useful in RA, although, like TGF-β, large amounts are already produced by the synovium.

C. Interfere with consequences of cytokines

The approaches previously outlined attempt to deal directly with cytokines, either by preventing production or interfering with their ability to signal cells. As an alternative strategy, one might choose to ignore these complex interactions, permit the cytokine network to rage unabated, and instead target specific deleterious effects of cytokines that contribute to disease perpetuation and morbidity. In RA, for instance, there are several potential cytokine actions that could be the focus of this strategy, such as 1) production of proteases involved in matrix destruction; 2) induction of adhesion molecules responsible for the recruitment and retention of inflammatory cells; and 3) production and regulation of a variety of secondary mediators, such as prostaglandins, leukotrienes, neuropeptides, bradykinin, etc., as well as other potentially important enzymes that are regulated by cytokines (e.g., phospholipase A2, COX2, and many others). The latter approach has a successful track record, with the non-steroidal anti-inflammatory drugs leading the way.

Perhaps of the most egregious weakness of current RA treatment is that joint destruction typically progresses despite symptomatic improvement (see Table 3). Hence, the inflammatory and destructive mechanisms of synovitis (especially in RA) appear to be quite distinct from each other.

Table 3.   Clinical effects of cyclo-oxygenase inhibitors

1.	Decreased morning stiffness
2.	Decreased swelling
3.	Decreased pain
4.	Variable or no effect on rheumatoid factor production
5.	No effect on cartilage loss
6.	No effect on progression of bone erosions

Matrix degradation is mediated by several families of proteolytic enzymes, including serine proteases, cysteine proteases, and metalloproteinases. It is not known which of these families is the most important in RA, although a great deal is understood about the regulation and distribution of the latter (17, 18). The primary source of collagenase and stromelysin is the synovial intimal lining, which is comprised of fibroblast-like and macrophage-like synoviocytes. Cytokines, especially IL-1 and TNF-α, are the major inducers of metalloproteinases in lining cells. Net tissue destruction results from excess metalloproteinase production compared to their natural inhibitors (known as TIMPs, or tissue inhibitors of metalloproteinases). While direct regulation of protease or TIMP gene expression through modulation of the cytokine network is desirable, it might be technically difficult. Instead, many investigators have elected to use more traditional medicinal chemistry approaches to develop small molecule inhibitors. In this paradigm, cytokines would continue to be synthesized and the enzymes produced; however, the ultimate destruction of cartilage, bone, and other connective tissues would be prevented.

This appealing approach does have some limitations. Like cytokines, a myriad of metalloproteinases are produced in the joint and the selection of one as the most important is difficult. Stromelysin is an attractive possibility, since it is abundant and has very broad substrate specificity. However, even if stromelysin is blocked by a specific inhibitor, there are dozens of other proteases that might extend matrix degradation. A second theoretical issue is that active collagenase and stromelysin are very difficult to detect in synovial fluid; they are almost exclusively present as inactive pro-enzymes or bound to TIMP. This observation is difficult to reconcile with current notions regarding the importance of metalloproteinases and suggests that these proteases are already inactivated almost as quickly as they are produced. The additional benefit of a competitive inhibitor under these circumstances is not known. A third obstacle is the fact that metalloproteinases play a role in normal homeostasis, wound healing, angiogenesis and other processes. Long term systemic inhibition might have unpredictable adverse effects.

While protease inhibitors are still relatively early in development, some encouraging data are available for cathepsin and collagenase inhibitors in animal models of adjuvant arthritis and collagen induced arthritis, respectively. These studies suggest that the joint destruction might be altered by blocking proteases, with both matrix protective effects and some surprising anti-inflammatory effects. They also support the notion that one might alter the natural history of disease by inhibiting only one of the many proteases present in the joint.

A second potential target for indirect "anti-cytokine" therapy is interference with cell trafficking in the synovium. This involves two distinct cytokine actions: 1) induction of adhesion molecules on endothelium by cytokines like IL-1 and TNF-α; and 2) promotion of cell migration into joint tissues by IL-8 and other chemokines. Inhibition of cell adhesion by blocking adhesion molecule function is under active clinical investigation. The most common strategies today include anti-ICAM-1 antibodies to block CD18 mediated binding and carbohydrates to interfere with selectin-mediated interactions. There is little published information on these approaches in long term models of arthritis, although there is a promising preliminary study in RA (19). However, there are many studies demonstrating the efficacy of anti-adhesion therapies in animal models of acute inflammation (20-23).

While development of small molecule competitive antagonists of adhesion proteins is only at an embryonic stage, other pharmacologic methods of interfering with cell adhesion are also feasible. For example, adenosine is known to inhibit neutrophil adhesion to activated endothelial cells. However, the therapeutic use of adenosine or other adenosine receptor agonists has been greatly limited by profound cardiovascular side effects. An alternative strategy might be to regulate adenosine production by cells in a site and event specific manner. Methotrexate, which is a commonly used agent in RA, appears to mediate some of its acute anti-inflammatory effects through this mechanism (24). However, its pharmacologic design as a folic acid antagonist and toxicity are probably unrelated to this mechanism. An example of a more direct approach to adenosine regulation is the development of specific inhibitors of enzymes involved in adenosine metabolism, such as adenosine kinase, a cytoplasmic enzyme that phosphorylates adenosine to AMP. In the presence of adenosine kinase inhibitors, adenosine release by activated endothelial cells is increased. Locally released adenosine can then bind to specific surface receptors on cells in the vicinity. Since the blood half life of adenosine is less than one second, the actions might be confined to its site of formation, thereby minimizing toxicity. Adenosine regulating agents block neutrophil adhesion to vascular endothelium in vitro and decrease neutrophil accumulation into inflamed sites in vivo (25).

VII. CONCLUSIONS

Understanding the cytokine profile of RA has recently altered the traditional view of synovitis. What began as a simple model of T cells orchestrating a local inflammatory response is now best regarded as a complex interplay between many cell types, each of which might predominate at various stages of the disease. The notion that antigen specific processes and local proliferation of lymphocytes account for articular T cell accumulation has been largely replaced by a concept in which antigen-independent signals, including chemokines and adhesion molecules, summon memory T cells into the joint. An unanswered question is "What do the T cells do after they enter the synovium?" Are a small percentage activated by an initiating or secondary antigen to perpetuate synovitis, or are they down regulating by suppressive factors in the joint? If they are not activated, then what maintains the chronic inflammatory response? One possibility is that transformed synoviocytes achieve a certain degree of autonomy. Or, perhaps a third cell type recently characterized and isolated from pannus (the "pannocyte") is a principle participant (26). In contemplating these issues, new therapeutic targets have been identified, with cytokine networks serving as a template for novel interventions.

VIII. REFERENCES

1.   Firestein GS, Xu WD, Townsend K, Broide D, Alvaro-Gracia J, Glasebrook A, et al. Cytokines in chronic inflammatory arthritis. 1. Failure to detect T cell lymphokines (IL-2 and IL-3) and presence of macrophage colony-stimulating factor (CSF-1) and a novel mast cell growth factor in rheumatoid synovitis. J Exp Med 1988; 168:1573-1586.

2.   Firestein GS, Zvaifler NJ. Peripheral blood and synovial fluid monocyte activation in inflammatory arthritis. II. Low levels of synovial fluid and synovial tissue interferon suggest that gamma-interferon is not the primary macrophage activating factor. Arthritis Rheum 1987; 30:864-8671.

3.   Miossec P, Naviliat M, Dupuy d'Angeac A, Banchereau JS. Low levels of interleukin-4 and high levels of transforming growth factor beta in rheumatoid arthritis. Arthritis Rheum. 1990; 145:2514-2519.

4.   Barnes PF, Fong SJ, Brennan PJ, Twomey PE, Mazumder A, Modin RL. Local production of tumor necrosis factor and IFN-γ in tuberculous pleuritis. 1990; J Immunol 145:149-154.

5.   Firestein GS, Zvaifler NJ. How important are T cells in chronic rheumatoid synovitis? Arthritis Rheum 1990; 33:768-773.

6.   Firestein GS, Alvaro-Gracia JM, Maki R. Quantitative analysis of cytokine gene expression in rheumatoid arthritis. J Immunol 1990; 144:3347-3353.

7.   Wahl SM, Allen JB, Wong HL, Dougherty SF, Ellingsworth LR. Antagonistic and agonistic effects of transforming growth factor-beta and IL-1 in rheumatoid synovitis. J Immunol 1990; 145:2514-2519.

8.   Katsikis PD, Chu CQ, Brennan FM, Maini RN, Feldmann M. Immunoregulatory role of interleukin 10 in rheumatoid arthritis. J Exp Med 1994; 179:1517-1527.

9.   Parmely MJ, Zhou WW, Edwards 3d CK, Borcherding DR, Silverstein R, Morrison DC. Adenosine and a related carbocyclic nucleoside analogue selectively inhibit tumor necrosis factor-alpha production and protect mice against endotoxin challenge. J Immunol 1993; 151:389-396.

10.   Williams RO, Mason LJ, Feldmann M, Maini RN. Synergy between anti-CD4 and anti-tumor necrosis factor in the amelioration of established collagen-induced arthritis. Proc Natl Acad Sci USA 1994; 91:2762-2766.

11.   Elliott MJ, Maini RN, Feldmann M, Long-Fox A, Charles P, Katsikis P, et al. Treatment of rheumatoid arthritis with chimeric monoclonal antibodies to tumor necrosis factor alpha. Arthritis Rheum 1993; 36:1681-1690.

12.   Eisenberg SP, Evans RJ, Arend WP, et al.. Primary structure and functional expression from complementary DNA of a human interleukin-1 receptor antagonist. Nature 1990; 343:341-346.

13.   Arend WP. Interleukin 1 receptor antagonist. A new member of the interleukin 1 family. J Clin Invest 1991; 88:1445-1451.

14. Alvaro-Gracia JM, Zvaifler NJ, Firestein GS. Cytokines in chronic inflammatory arthritis. V. Mutual antagonism between IFN-gamma and TNF-alpha on HLA-DR expression, proliferation, collagenase production, and GM-CSF production by rheumatoid arthritis synoviocytes. J Clin Invest 1990; 86:1790-1798.

15. Cannon GW, Emkey RD, Denes A, Cohen SA, Saway PA, Wolfe F, et al. Prospective two-year followup of recombinant interferon-gamma in rheumatoid arthritis. J Rheumatol 1990; 17:304-310.

16. Panitch HS, Bever CT Jr. Clinical trials of interferons in multiple sclerosis. What have we learned? J Neuroimmunol 1993; 46:155-164.

17. Woessner JF Jr. Matrix metalloproteinases and their inhibitors in connective tissue remodeling. FASEB J 1991; 5:2145-2154.

18. Firestein GS, Paine MM, Littman BH. Gene expression (collagenase, tissue inhibitor of metalloproteinases, complement, and HLA-DR) in rheumatoid arthritis and osteoarthritis synovium: Quantitative analysis and effect of intraarticular corticosteroids. Arthritis Rheum 1994; 34:1094-1105.

19. Kavanaugh AF, Laurie SD, Nichols LA, Norris SH, Rothlein R, Scharschmidt LA, et al. Treatment of refractory rheumatoid arthritis with a monoclonal antibody to intercellular adhesion molecule 1. J Immunol 1994, 37:992-999.

20. Mulligan MS, Varani J, Warren JS, Till GO, Smith CW, Anderson DC, et al. Roles of $\beta 2$ integrins of rat neutrophils in complement- and oxygen radical-mediated acute inflammatory injury. J Immunol 1992; 148:1847-1857.

21. Thomas JR, Harlan JM, Rice CL, Winn RK. Role of leukocyte CD11/CD18 complex in endotoxic and septic shock in rabbits. J Appl Physiol 1992; 73:1510-1516.

22. Walsh CJ, Carey PD, Cook DJ, Bechard DE, Fowler AA, Sugerman HJ. Anti-CD18 antibody attenuates, neutropenia and alveolar capillary-membrane. Surgery 1991; 110:205-212.

23. Mulligan MS, Polley MJ, Bayer RJ, Nunn MF, Paulson JC, Ward PA. Neutrophil-dependent acute lung injury: requirement for P-selectin (GMP-140). J Clin Invest 1992; 90:1600-1607.

24. Cronstein BN, Naime D, Ostad E. The antiinflammatory mechanism of methotrexate. Increased adenosine release at inflamed sites diminishes leukocyte accumulation in an in vivo model of inflammation. J Clin Invest 1993; 92:2675-2682.

25. Firestein GS, Boyle D, Bullough DA, Gruber HE, Sajjadi FG, Montag A, et al. Protective effect of an adenosine kinase inhibitor in septic shock. J Immunol 1994; 152:5853-5859.

26. Zvaifler NJ, Firestein GS. Pannus and pannocytes. Alternative models of joint destruction in rheumatoid arthritis. Arthritis Rheum 1994; 37:783-9.

AAS 47
Inflammation:
Mechanisms and Therapeutics
© 1995 Birkhäuser Verlag Basel

T CELL RECEPTOR PEPTIDE VACCINES AS IMMUNOTHERAPY

Steven W. Brostoff

The Immune Response Corporation
5935 Darwin Court, Carlsbad, CA 92008, USA

Many of the major autoimmune diseases, such as rheumatoid arthritis, multiple sclerosis, psoriasis and Type 1 diabetes, are considered to be T cell-mediated diseases. Since T cells are responsible for the tissue damage in these diseases, these autoreactive T cells can be characterized as pathogens. Common pathogens, such as viruses and bacteria, can be controlled by vaccines comprised of killed or attenuated pathogens or subunits of these pathogens. In the case of autoreactive T cell pathogens, a killed or attenuated vaccine approach can be used (1), but would have little appeal as a viable, commercial product because individual differences in transplantation antigens would require it to be given as an autologous vaccine. T cells from each patient would have to be removed from the body, killed or attenuated and then reinfused back into the patient. Such a procedure would be very costly, time consuming and inefficient. However, a subunit type of therapeutic could be practical. The subunit of the T cell that distinguishes one T cell from another, and therefore distinguishes the pathogenic T cells from the normal T cells, is the T cell receptor. A vaccination approach involving the T cell receptor as a subunit is appealing, not only because of its specificity, but because of the opportunity it affords to produce a long lasting immunoregulation, which contrasts with other approaches utilizing monoclonal antibodies, drugs that block the MHC or anti-inflammatories that treat symptoms without affecting the underlying disease process. Targeting T cell receptors on autoreactive T cells requires that the T cell receptor repertoire be sufficiently restricted in any particular disease in order to increase the feasibility of this approach.

The animal model of experimental autoimmune encephalomyelitis has been an important tool for studying T cell-mediated autoimmune disease and developing therapeutic strategies for treating such diseases. In addition, studies using this model have proven useful in understanding immunoregulation (2). Restricted T cell receptor gene usage in autoimmune disease was first noted in this animal model (3-6) and led to the development of T cell receptor peptide immunization as a means to control autoimmune disease (7, 8).

T cells that cause experimental autoimmune encephalomyelitis in mice and rats use a limited number of T cell receptor gene elements (2-6). Despite differences in the MHC-restricting elements, the T cells causing encephalomyelitis in PL/J mice, B10.PL mice and Lewis rats all are dominated by the use of the Vß8.2 gene element. Injection of peptides from the CDR2 or CDR3 Vß8.2 region has proven useful in preventing the clinical manifestations of this disease (7, 8). Such success with animal models led directly to the search for restricted T cell receptor gene use in human autoimmune disease. Early reports indicated that rheumatoid arthritis (9, 10) and multiple sclerosis (11-13) were restricted in their T cell receptor gene use. Our studies in rheumatoid arthritis (10) showed that the majority of activated T cells infiltrating synovial tissue in rheumatoid arthritis patients over-utilized Vß3, Vß14 and Vß17. Moreover, T cells containing these Vßs that infiltrated synovial tissue were dominated by one or a few clones indicating that clonal expansion *in situ* in response to a tissue antigen had taken place.

Moreover, the close relationships of the three Vßs found implicated superantigen in the disease process, since these three Vßs are closely related in the fourth hypervariable region known to bind superantigen. Superantigens are so named because they stimulate large subsets of T cells non-specifically (i.e., independent of nominal antigen) by binding T cell receptor and MHC outside of the peptide binding groove, resulting in the stimulation of all T cells bearing selected Vßs (14). Superantigens are usually products of virus or bacteria. One scenario for the role of superantigens in the pathogenesis of autoimmune disease (14) is for such antigens to be released into a host organism systemically after a bacterial or viral infection. These superantigens could then stimulate potentially autoreactive T cells which had escaped deletion during development. Such non-specifically stimulated T cells would then locate their target antigens and expand and attack the target tissue in response to autoantigen. Evidence that the infiltrating T cells are dominated by only one or a few clones suggest that the target of autoreactive T cells is tissue antigen rather than an endogenous superantigen localized in the target tissue since the latter would lead to a polyclonal population of T cells utilizing a given Vß.

In collaboration with the Psoriasis Research Institute (Palo Alto, CA), we have also found evidence of restricted Vß gene use in psoriasis (15). Psoriasis is an inflammatory skin disorder characterized by epidermal keratinocyte hyperproliferation in association with a cellular infiltrate. Because psoriasis has HLA class I association, restriction in the Vß gene use among CD8$^+$ T cells in psoriatic lesions might be expected. We examined the T cell receptor Vß gene use of epidermal CD8$^+$ and CD4$^+$ T cells in shave biopsies of psoriatic lesions. Our results show an elevated skin (over PBL) expression of Vß3 and/or Vß13.1 messages in the CD8$^+$, but not the CD4$^+$, T cells in a majority of patients studied. CDR3 sequence analysis on these two Vßs from the skin demonstrated monoclonality or marked oligoclonality. A second biopsy performed 3.5 to 8 months later in 4 patients, at the same or different lesions, again revealed an elevated Vß3 and/or Vß13.1 expression and clonality. Moreover, in three of the four patients, the same T cell receptor Vß CDR3 rearrangement was found in both biopsies. The persistence of Vß3 and/or Vß13.1-bearing CD8$^+$ T cells in lesions that did not undergo resolution suggests their role as effector cells rather than as regulatory cells. It is interesting to note that a superantigen from *Yersinia pseudotuberculosis* has recently been reported to stimulate both Vß3 and Vß13.1 T cells (16, 17).

Since immunization with T cell receptor peptides has proven useful in controlling animal models of autoimmune disease, we sought to apply such an approach to treatment of human autoimmune disease (18). Following our observation that Vß17 was over utilized in rheumatoid arthritis, we initiated a phase I open-label safety and dose-ranging study (in collaboration with The University of Alabama, Birmingham, and the Sharp Rees-Steely Medical Group in San Diego) to investigate the feasibility of T cell receptor peptide immunization as therapy for rheumatoid arthritis. The purpose of this initial study was to establish safety, optimal dose and biologic effects of immunization with varying doses of a 17 amino acid sequence derived from the CDR2 region of the human Vß17 T cell receptor. Fifteen moderate to severe rheumatoid arthritis patients received an intramuscular injection of one of four doses of the peptide in incomplete Freund's adjuvant, followed by a booster injection of the same dose of peptide four weeks later. The doses given were 10 μg, 30 μg, 100 μg and 300 μg. Patients were followed for 48 weeks post immunization to monitor for safety. Nonblinded assessment of disease, measured by number of swollen and tender joints, showed trends towards improvement over the

48 week follow-up period. In addition to safety measurements, a variety of immunogenicity measurements were used to measure the effect, if any, of the immunization on the immune system and the target Vß17 T cell population. Significant T cell proliferation in response to the immunizing Vß17 peptide was observed at 6 weeks or later post-immunization in a subset of patients. Percentages of activated Vß17 T cells in peripheral blood of patients in the highest dose groups (100 μg and 300 μg) were also measured post-immunization. The majority of these patients showed a reduction in activated Vß17 T cells in the peripheral blood. The T cell receptor peptide immunization appeared to be safe and well-tolerated. No significant adverse events attributable to the treatment were experienced. Further studies will be required to assess the significance of the biologic effects observed post immunization and a double-blind controlled trial will be needed to assess efficacy of this treatment approach.

REFERENCES

1. Ben-Nun A, Wekerle H, Cohen IR. Vaccination against autoimmune encephalomyelitis with T-lymphocyte line cells reactive against myelin basic protein. Nature 1981; 292:60-61.

2. Wraith DC, McDevitt HO, Steinman L, Acha-Orbea H. T cell recognition as the target for immune intervention in autoimmune disease. Cell 1989; 57-709-715.

3. Acha-Orbea H, Mitchell DJ, Timmermann L, Wraith DC, Tausch GS, Waldor MK, Zamvil SS, McDevitt HO, Steinman L. Limited heterogeneity of T cell receptors from lymphocytes mediating autoimmune encephalomyelitis allows specific immune intervention. Cell 1988; 54:263-273.

4. Urban JL, Kumar V, Kono DH, Gomez C, Horvath SJ, Clayton J, Ando DG, Sercarz EE, Hood L. Restricted use of T cell receptor V genes in murine autoimmune encephalomyelitis raises possibilities for antibody therapy. Cell 1988; 54:577-592.

5. Burns FR, Li X, Shen N, Offner H, Chou YK, Vandenbark AA, Herber-Katz E. Both rat and mouse T cell receptors specific for the encephalitogenic determinants of myelin basic protein use similar Vα or Vß chain genes even though the major histocompatibility complex and encephalitogenic determinants being recognized are different. J Exp Med 1989; 169:27-39.

6. Chluba J, Steeg C, Becker A, Wekerle H, Epplen JT. T cell receptor ß chain usage in myelin basic protein-specific rat T lymphocytes. Eur J Immunol 1989; 19:279-284.

7. Howell MD, Winters ST, Olee T, Powell HC, Carlo DJ, Brostoff SW. Vaccination against experimental allergic encephalomyelitis with T cell receptor peptides. Science 1989; 246:668-670.

8. Vandenbark AA, Hashim G, Offner H. Immunization with a synthetic T-cell receptor V-region peptide protects against experimental autoimmune encephalomyelitis. Nature 1989; 341:541-544.

9. Paliard X, West SG, Lafferty JA, Clements JR, Kappler JW, Marrack P, Kotzin BL. Evidence for the effects of a superantigen in rheumatoid arthritis. Science 1991; 253:325-329.

10. Howell MD, Diveley JP, Lundeen KA, Esty A, Winters ST, Carlo DJ, Brostoff SW. Limited T cell receptor ß-chain heterogeneity among IL-2R+ synovial T cells suggests a role for superantigen in rheumatoid arthritis. PNAS 1991; 88:10921-10925.

11. Oksenberg JR, Stuart S, Begovich AB, Bell RB, Erlich HA, Steinman L, Bernard CCA. Limited heterogeneity of rearranged T-cell receptor Vα transcripts in brains of multiple sclerosis patients. Nature 1990; 345:344-346.

12. Wucherpfennig KW, Ota K, Endo N, Seidman JG, Roxenzweig A, Weiner HL, Hafler DA. Shared human T cell receptor Vß usage to immunodominant regions of myelin basic protein. Science 1990; 248:1016-1019.

13. Lee SJ, Wucherpfennig KW, Brod SA, Benjamin D, Weiner HL, Hafler DA. Common T-cell receptor Vß usage in oligoclonal T lymphocytes derived from cerebrospinal fluid and blood of patients with multiple sclerosis. Ann Neurol 1991; 29:33-39.

14. Marrack P, Kappler J. The staphylococcal enterotoxins and their relatives. Science 1990; 248:705.

15. Chang JCC, Smith LR, Froning KJ, Schwabe BJ, Laxer JA, Caralli LL, Kurland HH, Karasek MA, Wilkinson DI, Carlo DJ, Brostoff SW. CD8+ T Cells in Psoriatic Lesions Preferentially Use T Cell Receptors Vß3 and/or Vß13.1 Genes. Proc Nat Acad Sci USA 1994; 91:9282-9286.

16. Abe J, Takeda T, Watanabe Y, Nakao H, Kobayashi N, Leung DYM, Kohsaka T. Evidence for superantigen production by Yersinia pseudotuberculosis. J Immunol 1993; 151:4183-4188.

17. Uchiyama T, Miyoshi-Akiyama T, Kato H, Fugimaki W, Imanishi K, Yan X-J. Superantigenic properties of a novel mitogenic substance produced by Yersinia pseudotuberculosis isolated from patients manifesting acute systemic symptoms. J Immunol 1993; 151:4407-4413.

18. Moreland LW, Heck LW Jr, Koopman WJ, Saway PA, Adamson TC, Fronek Z, O'Connor RD, Morgan EE, Diveley JP, Chieffo NM, Freeman TD, Carlo DJ, Brostoff SW. Vß17 T Cell Receptor Peptide Vaccine: Results of a Phase I Dose-Finding Study in Patients with Rheumatoid Arthritis. Ann. NY Acad. Sci. USA 1994; (in press).

AAS 47
Inflammation:
Mechanisms and Therapeutics
© 1995 Birkhäuser Verlag Basel

ANTIGEN SPECIFIC THERAPIES FOR THE TREATMENT OF AUTOIMMUNE DISEASES

David A. Hafler [1] and Howard L. Weiner[2]

[1]Laboratory of Molecular Immunology and [2]The MS Clinical and Research Unit,
Center for Neurologic Diseases, Brigham & Women's Hospital
and
Harvard Medical School, Boston MA 02115

OVERVIEW OF HUMAN AUTOIMMUNE DISEASE

Disease initiation. There are two general hypotheses for the etiology of human autoimmune disorders. In the first instance, the organ becomes infected by a virus or other infectious agent and cells that infiltrate that organ are targeted to the infectious agent. These events would then begin the cascade leading to the organ specific autoimmune disease. The alternative hypothesis is that the initial infiltrating cells are autoimmune in nature and recognize the organ specific proteins that are presented by local antigen presenting cells in the context of MHC. At our present state of knowledge, either hypothesis is possible. However, once the autoimmune cascade begins it is likely that "epitope spreading" will occur, and T cells recognizing other organ speicifc proteins will be recruited. Perhaps viruses and infectious agents acting as superantigens initially trigger or drive the autoimmune process, as opposed to being the primary target of infiltrating cells. Understanding the mechanism for initiation of autoimmune disorders and the range of antigens recognized by self-reactive T cells is critical for developing antigen specific therapies for these disorders.

Organ Specific Proteins as Targets for T Cells. What are the characteristics of a tissue specific autoantigen that will be recognized by T cells? Approximately 0.1% of a restricting class II MHC protein must be occupied with the antigen peptide for T cell activation to occur (1). Considering there is competition by a large variety of self and foreign peptides for binding to MHC class II proteins (2), it is possible that this requirement may be met only by peptides which are present in relatively large quantities in antigen presenting cells, processed efficiently and bound with a high affinity to class II molecules. Thus, the physical characteristics and processing of the antigen in the tissue may limit the number of potential autoantigens that the immune system is capable of recognizing.

Secondly, a T cell autoantigen must be processed in such a way as to be presented by class II MHC by the antigen presenting cells specific for that tissue site (Fig. 1). Using the central nervous system as an example, microglia, which are specialized CNS macrophages, might phagocytose breakdown products of myelin and present peptide antigens to T cells (3, 4). Alternatively, glial cells such as astrocytes, which after activation can express class II MHC and present antigen, might present CNS antigens in the context of class II MHC (5, 6).

Epitope mapping of autoantigen. Of the central nervous system antigens, myelin basic protein (MBP) is perhaps the most extensively characterized autoantigens and is a primary candidate autoantigen in MS because of its ability to induce EAE. We will use MBP as an example in discussing epitope mapping. There have been many investigations of MBP reactivity in MS using seven day proliferation assays of whole peripheral blood mononuclear cells (7, 8). These investigations have shown a slight increase in T cell responses to human MBP in subjects with MS as compared to normal subjects or other neurologic disease patients, but the magnitude of the difference has generally been less than convincing. T cell cloning techniques have recently been applied to study autoreactive T cells both in the peripheral blood and spinal fluid. Antigen specific T cell clones are generated by repeated stimulation and culture of T cells with antigen in the presence of T cell growth factors.

In the EAE model, T cell clones can be derived from animals injected with MBP in adjuvant that recognize immunodominant regions of MBP that are influenced by the MHC of the animal. These clones can transfer EAE when injected into naive animals (9-12). For example in Lewis rats, the MBP(68-88) peptide is immunodominant and is the epitope for the majority of encephalitogenic T cell clones (10-12). Lewis rat T cell clones generated against MBP (residues 43-67) are only weakly able to cause disease.

In humans, immunodominant regions of MBP that are presented by defined MHC proteins have beeen identifed. Immunodominant regions of MBP are between residues 84-106 and 143-172 near the C terminus (13-17) . In DR2+ individuals, a high proportion of T cell clones reactive with MBP recognized the 84-106 region, whether or not they had MS (13). Both DR and DQ antigens were found to be reestricting elements indicating that immunodominant MBP peptides can be presented by different class II molecules. It has also been demonstrated that T cells from genetically diverse individuals responding to different epitopes of human MBP are associated with distinct MHC class II molecules (18). Of interest was the finding that DR2+

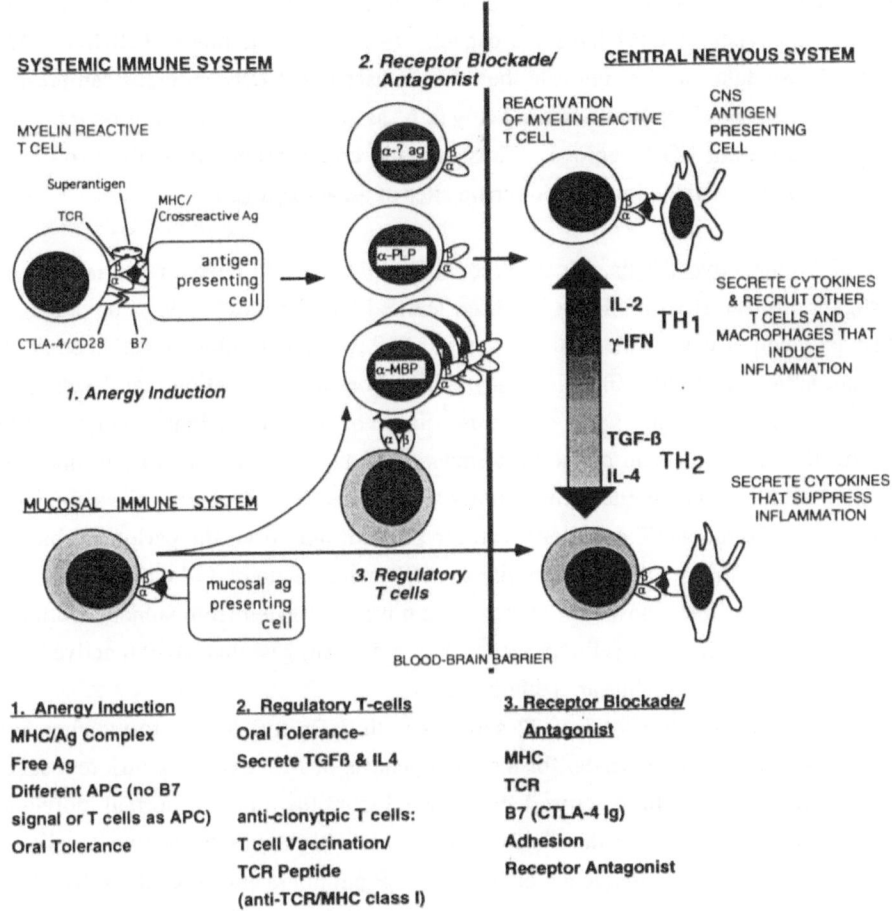

Figure 1. Overview of proposed pathophysiology for MS and specific areas where immune system can be manipulated. The minimal requirements in mammals for inducing inflammatory autoimmune disease in the CNS white matter are activated CD4+ T cells recognizing MBP or PLP. In MS, we hypothesize that some activating event, such as a viral superantigen or molecular mimicry activates an autoreactive T cell. This allows the activate T cell to migrate into the CNS where it can now recognize CNS antigen in the context of MHC, recruiting effector cells leading to the inflammatory CNS response. The process may be blocked by 1). Anergy induction; 2) By regulatory T cells; or 3) by receptor blockade or antagonist (see text).

possessed an unusual capacity to restrict all of the epitopes identified on MBP (15, 16, 18). Moreover, different types of DR2 have the capacity to present a number of different MBP epitopes (19). These data together indicate that disease associated DR2 antigens can present a variety of MBP peptides to T cells and this is likely to be associated with competition for peptide binding between different MBP regions. Thus, peptide competition for binding to class II molecules may in part determine immunodominant sites of an autoantigen.

Activation of Autoreactive T cells. T cells recognizing MBP and PLP exist in normal humans. From investigation of the EAE model, it has been learned that for these cells to be pathogenic they must be activated *in vivo*. To examine whether MBP reactive T cells are activated *in vivo*, an hprt⁻ mutant assay was used (20). The assay is based on the observation that dividing cells acquire random mutations during DNA synthesis. Some of these mutations occur in the hprt gene which results in inactivation of the hprt enzyme. Thus, mutant cells do not metabolize thioguanine to a cytotoxic metabolite, which allows a very effective selection of these mutants in culture. Eleven of 258 mutant T cell clones cultured by mitogen from the peripheral blood of five of six MS patients showed strong reactivity to MBP, while none of 114 clones grown from blood of normal subjects did. However, clones were not investigated from subjects with other neurologic diseases or with non-myelin antigens. These data suggest that MBP reactive T cells are activated in MS patients and thus are pathogenic.

We directly investigated in a total of 72 subjects with definitive MS as to whether myelin reactive T cells, which might be critical for the pathogenesis of MS, exist in a different state of activation as compared to myelin reactive T cells cloned from the blood of normal individuals. While there were no differences in the the frequencies of MBP and PLP-reactive T cells after primary antigen stimulation, the frequency of MBP or PLP but not tetanus toxoid reactive T cells generated after primary rIL-2 stimulation was significantly higher in MS patients as compared to control individuals. Primary rIL-2 stimulated MBP-reactive T cell lines were CD4+, and recognized MBP epitopes 84-102 and 143-168 similar to MBP-reactive T cell lines generated with primary MBP stimulation. In the CSF of MS patients, MBP-reactive T cells generated with primary rIL-2 stimulation accounted for 7% of the IL-2 responsive cells, greater than 10-fold higher than paired blood samples, and these T cells also selectively recognized MBP peptides 84-102 and 143-168. In striking contrast, MBP-reactive T cells were not detected in CSF obtained from patients with other neurologic diseases. These results provide definitive *in vitro* evidence of an absolute difference in the activation state of myelin reactive T cells in the central nervous system of patients with MS, and provide evidence of a pathogenic role of autoreactive T cells in the disease.

If circulating, autoreactive T cells are present in the circulation of normal individuals, how do they become activated (Fig. 1)? The mechanism is of particular interest in a CNS disease such as MS, since resting T cells appear unable to cross the blood-brain barrier. Possible mechanisms in the absence of autoantigen involve immune activation associated with infections which include: 1) molecular mimicry, 2) activation by superantigens, and 3) bystander CD2 activation.

ORAL TOLERANCE; ANTIGEN SPECIFIC IMMUNOTHERAPY

Overview of Antigen Specific Immunotherapy. In the section above, we presented an overview of antigen specific recognition in autoimmune diseases. In total, these experiments suggest a number of manipulations that may be used to block the immune response. It is important to note the liklihood that no *in vitro* experiment can prove the autoimmune hypothesis for any of the presumed autoimmune diseases. Instead, only specific manipulations *in vivo* where antigen reactive cells are targeted with associated amelioration of disease activity will allow the understanding of the disease's pathogenesis. Thus, these specific manipulations of the immune response represent both attempts to treat the disease as well as scientific experiments to undertand the disease.

There are two general aproaches to antigen specific immunotherapy of autoimmune disease. One approach is to block either the initial activation or the subsequent recognition of autoantigen by autoreactive T cells (see Fig. 1). This approach requires the immune response against the self-antigen to be restricted in terms of either the number of epitopes recognized or the TCR repertoire that is used. This includes MHC blocking peptides, TCR antagonists, and TCR peptides which may inhibit specific T cell function. Using MS as an example, it would appear that although there are MBP and PLP dominant epitopes and somewhat restricted use of TCRs in their recognition, the outbred human species contains too many myelin reactive T cells with different TCR usage to sucessfully inhibit the total of the spreading immune response to myelin antigens.

The second approach involves the antigen specific targeting of T cells that downregulate immune responses to the inflammatory sites. In this instance, it is not necessary to know the inciting antigen that elicites the immune response nor is it required that the T cells be restricted in terms of antigen recognition or TCR usage. This approach may well be be physiologic in regulating the normal immune response. One such method which has attracted much attention recently is the use of oral tolerization, where the autoantigen is delivered orally with the generation of T cells secreting TGF-ß, IL-4, and IL-10 that migrate to the site of inflammation and suppress the immune response.

Mechanism of Oral Tolerance. Oral tolerance represents the exogenous administration of antigen to the peripheral immune system via the gut. As such, it is a form of antigen-driven peripheral immune tolerance. Immunologic tolerance is not programmed into the germ line but is acquired during maturation of the immune system by mechanisms that delete or inactivate antigen-reactive clones. There are three basic mechanisms to explain antigen-driven tolerance: clonal deletion, clonal anergy, and active suppression (21, 22). A large number of studies have shown that one of the primary mechanims associated with oral tolerance is the generation of active suppression (23). More recently, clonal anergy has been demonstrated (24, 25). There is little evidence that orally administered antigen induces clonal deletion. During the course of our investigations we have delineated two pathways by which oral tolerization results in systemic hyporesponsiveness by either active suppression or clonal anergy (26). These pathways are described below in a schema which forms the theoretical basis for this review.

Based on recent findings in our laboratory and others, we believe that oral tolerance can be viewed as anergy-driven oral tolerance or regulatory-cell-driven oral tolerance. The primary factor which determines which form of peripheral tolerance develops following oral administration of antigen is the dose of antigen fed. Low doses of antigen favor the generation of active suppression or regulatory-cell driven tolerance whereas high doses of antigen favor anergy-driven tolerance (Fig. 2). Although these forms of oral tolerance are not mutually exclusive and may occur simultaneously, they are distinct and the use of oral tolerance to treat autoimmune diseases is critically dependent on which of these two mechanisms is triggered.

The delineation of these two mechanisms of oral tolerance was based on the following: 1) Investigations in our laboratory using low doses of orally administered autoantigens were shown to suppress experimental autoimmune diseases via the generation of regulatory cells that suppressed *in vitro* and *in vivo* via the secretion of downregulatory cytokines such as TGFb (27); 2) Investigations from other laboratories which demonstrated clonal anergy following oral administration of large doses of antigen with no evidence of active suppression (24, 25); 3) A large series of investigations demonstrated transferrable suppression following oral tolerance including work which showed two components of oral tolerance, one that was abrogated by treatment with low dose cyclophosphamide and one that was not, a difference that was dose dependent (28); and 4) Direct comparison in our laboratory demonstrating that the two mechanisms depend on the dose (26)(Fig. 2).

As shown in Fig. 2, low doses of antigen result in the generation of antigen specific regulatory cells, and as such involve presentation of antigen by gut-associated antigen presenting cells. Such presentation preferentially induces regulatory cells which upon subsequent recognition of antigen *in vivo* or *in vitro*, secrete the suppressive cytokine TGFb. In addition,

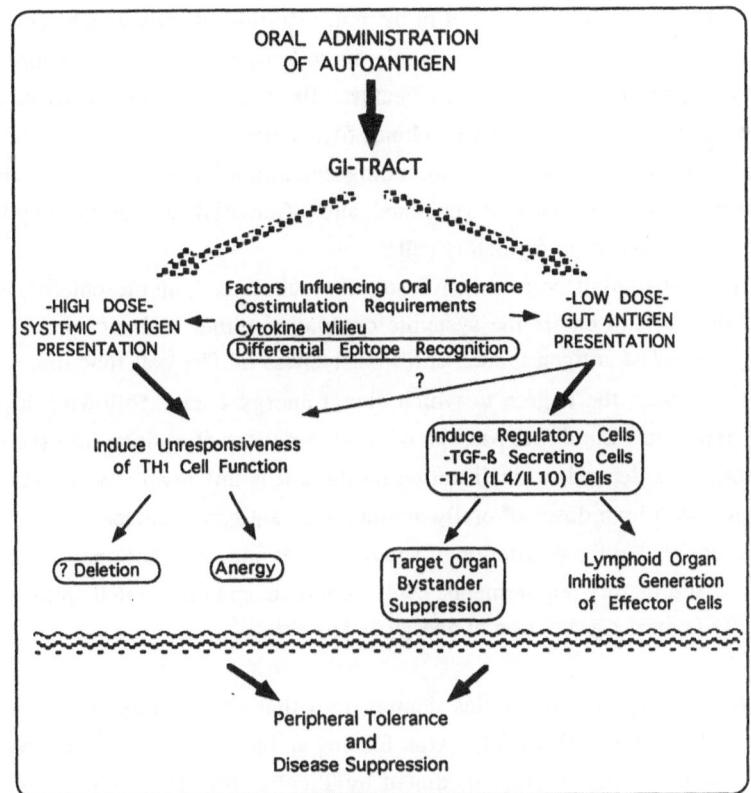

Figure 2. Mechanisms of oral tolerance
High dose antigen administration leads to the generation of anergy, while lower dose oral antigen induces regulatory T cells that secrete TGFß1 and/or IL-4/IL-10 which migrate to the CNS and down regulate the local immune response.

Th2 responses are preferentially generated in the gut, resulting in cells which secrete IL-4 and IL-10. These antigen specific regulatorycells migrate to lymphoid organs and suppress immune responses by inhibiting the generation of effector cells, and to the target organ to suppress disease by releasing antigen non-specific cytokines (bystander suppression). Several factors can affect the generation of regulatory cells including costimulation requirements, the cytokine milieu in which the immune response is generated, and differential generation of epitopes which preferentially may trigger certain regulatory cells.

High doses of orally administered antigen result in systemic antigen presentation after antigen passes through the gut and enters the systemic circulation either as intact protein or antigen fragments. High doses of antigen induce unresponsiveness of Th1 cell function, primarily via clonal anergy. Whether, the degree to which clonal anergy occurs following high doses of antigen merely represents the direct passage of small amounts of antigen into the systemic or portal circulation, or is dependent on filtration by the gut is unknown. Why there is reduced active suppression with high doses of orally administered antigen is unclear, but could relate to anergizing cells involved in the generation of active suppression. In addition, it is not known the degree to which costimulatory requirements, cytokine milieu, and differential epitope recognition may preferentially favor the generation of anergy in Th1 cells.

Active Suppression. Many studies demonstrate that active suppression is an important mechanism for oral tolerance (23, 29-34). After feeding antigens such as ovalbumin or sheep red blood cells, transferrable suppression mediated by T cells from Peyer's patches, mesenteric lymph node, and spleen has been demonstrated. Investigators have also reported initial sensitization prior to the appearance of suppression (30). Further characterization of active suppression as measured in these systems has not occurred, most probably related to the difficulties in defining the biology of suppression (35, 36). Nonetheless the demonstration of transferrable cellular suppression associated with oral tolerance is a recurrent theme reported by many investigators (23).

Our studies of oral tolerance in autoimmune models have found active suppression to be a primary mechanism and have identified regulatory cells generated following oral tolerance which act via the secretion to antigen-nonspecific downregulatory cytokines following triggering by the fed antigen (37). These cells have been characterized both in the rat and murine model of EAE orally tolerized to MBP. In the Lewis rat model, regulatory cells were CD8+ (38), and acted via the secretion of TGFb following antigen specific triggering (27). They transfer suppression *in vivo* and can suppress *in vitro*. The epitopes of guinea pig MBP triggering CD8+ regulatory cells following orally administered MBP were different than the encephalitogenic determinant (39). In addition, TGFb-secreting regulatory cells can be found in Peyer's patches 24-48 hours after one feeding of MBP (40). Of note is that cells from Peyer's patches removed after one feeding of MBP do not proliferate in response to MBP even though they release TGFb upon *in vitro* stimulation. The mechanism by which these regulatory cells are induced remains unknown. It is also not known the degree to which the generation of regulatory cells is related to unique antigen-presenting cells in the gut, the cytokine milieu, or other factors. Using murine models of oral tolerance suggest that in addition to CD8+ TGFb secreting regulatory cells, CD4+ regulatory cells are also induced. These CD4+ cells secrete IL-4 and IL-10 in addition to TGFb. Moreover, these TGFß secreting T cells can adoptively transfer suppression of EAE to naive animals (41).

Anergy. Anergy has only recently been demonstrated as a possible mechanism for oral tolerance (24, 25). Anergy is defined as a state of T lymphocyte unresponsiveness characterized by absence of proliferation, IL-2 production and diminished expression of IL-2R (42). Anergy may be experimentally differentiated from clonal deletion by demonstrating the presence of antigen specific TcR clonotypes, or by release from the anergic state which is accomplished by pre-culture of cells in IL-2 (43). Under these conditions we have shown that a single feeding of 20 mg OVA induced a state of anergy in OVA specific T lymphocytes: cells did not respond to OVA by proliferation, OVA stimulation did not induce IL-2 production or IL2R expression, and the non-responsive state was reversed by pre-culture of tolerized cells in IL-2 (25). One other study has indirectly demonstrated anergy as a mechanism for oral tolerance (24). Whitacre et al. reported diminished IL-2 and IFN-g production in rats orally fed MBP in the presence of the soybean protease inhibitor; however, anergy was not confirmed in this study by TcR analysis or by IL-2 driven release. As discussed previously, the induction of anergy depends upon antigen dosage and frequency of feeding (26).

TREATMENT OF ORGAN SPECIFIC AUTOIMMUNE DISEASES IN ANIMALS

We have examined the manner in which oral tolerance may be applied to the treatment of autoimmune conditions in both humans and animals. Thompson and Staines (44) and Nagler-Anderson, et al.,(45) initially described suppression of collagen induced arthritis by feeding type II collagen. Our laboratory (46-48) and that of Whitacre's (24, 49, 50) have studied suppression of EAE by orally administered myelin antigens. Additionally, we have investigated oral tolerance to suppress autoimmune models of uveitis, (51) diabetes in the NOD mouse (52, 53) and adjuvant arthritis (54, 55), as well as orally-administered alloantigen or MHC peptide in transplantation models (56-58).

Investigators have also demonstrated suppression of other autoimmune models by orally administered antigen (59). Thus, the ability to suppress autoimmunity in animal models via oral tolerance has been established although the mechanisms responsible may differ depending on the laboratory and the models being studied.

EAE. Orally-administered guinea pig MBP suppresses EAE in the Lewis rat model (46, 49). As discussed above, this effect is mediated both by actve suppression and anergy. An important question before entering human clinical trials was whether or not ongoing disease could be suppressed. We investigated chronic relapsing EAE in the Lewis rat and strain 13 guinea pig. Disease was also suppressed by oral administration of MBP or a bovine myelin preparation that is also being administered in human clinical trials. There was no exacerbation of disease in these animals, demonstrating that orally administered antigens do not appear to prime rather than suppress in an already immunized animal. Of note in the guinea pig model is that 10 mg of bovine myelin fed 3 times per week over a 3 month period suppressed disease and histologic manifestations, whereas feeding 50 mg of bovine myelin did not. This may indicate that bystander suppression was responsible for the effect on chronic disease, and that in some instances, the oral administration of too high a dose will not suppress autoimmune models. As discussed later, loss of protection by orally administered antigen at higher doses was also seen with orally-administered collagen in adjuvant arthritis and orally-administered insulin to suppress diabetes in the NOD mouse.

Lastly, we will discuss the immunohistology associated with oral tolerization to MBP and in animals naturally recovering from EAE (56). Brains from OVA fed animals at the peak of disease showed perivascular infiltration with activated mononuclear cells which secreted the inflammatory cytokines ILl, IL-2, TNF-a, IFN-g, IL-6 and IL-8. Inhibitory cytokines, TGF-b and IL-4, and prostaglandin E_2 (PGE$_2$) were absent. In MBP orally tolerized animals, there was a marked reduction of the perivascular infiltrate and down regulation of all inflammatory cytokines. In addition, there was up regulation of the inhibitory cytokine TGF-b. When bacterial lipopolysaccharide (LPS) was fed in addition to MBP, protection against EAE was enhanced and was associated with elevated IL-4 and PGE$_2$ in the brain (56, 60). In control recovering animals (day 18) staining for inflammatory cytokines was diminished and there was upregulation of TGF-b and IL-4. These results suggest that the suppression of EAE by oral tolerization and natural recovery is related to regulatory cells that secrete inhibitory cytokines at the target organ.

Collagen and Adjuvant Arthritis. Previous investigators have demonstrated suppression of collagen-induced arthritis by feeding collagen type II (44,45) We have studied adjuvant arthritis (AA) in the rat, a well-characterized and more fulminant form of experimental arthritis (54). Oral administration of chicken collagen type II (CII), given at a dose of 3 mg per feeding, consistently suppressed the development of AA. A decrease in DTH responses to CII was observed that correlated with suppression to AA. Oral administration of collagen type I also suppressed AA; only minimal effects were seen with collagen type III. Suppression was antigen specific in that feeding collagen type II did not suppress EAE, and feeding MBP did not suppress AA. Suppression of AA could be adoptively transferred by T cells from CII-fed animals and was observed when CII was fed after disease onset. Of note is that suppression was observed at doses of 3 and 30 mg, but not at 300 or 1000 mg. These results suggest that oral collagen is suppressing AA via bystander suppression rather than clonal anergy since active suppression may be lost at higher doses. The effectiveness of such small amounts of oral collagen may be related to the fact that collagen has repeating amino acid subunits.

Uveitis. Oral administration of S-antigen (S-Ag), a retinal autoantigen that induces experimental autoimmune uveitis (EAU), prevented or markedly diminished the clinical appearance of S-Ag-induced disease as measured by ocular inflammation (51, 61-66). Furthermore, oral administration of S-Ag also markedly diminished uveitis induced by the uveitogenic M and N fragments of the S-Ag. Oral administration of S-Ag did not prevent MBP-induced EAE. In vitro studies demonstrated a significant decrease in proliferative responses to the S-Ag in lymph node cells draining the site of immunization from fed versus nonfed animals. Furthermore, the addition of splenocytes from S-Ag-fed animals to cultures of a CD4$^+$ S-Ag-specific lymphocyte line profoundly suppressed the line's response to the S-Ag, whereas these splenocytes had no effect on a PPD-specific lymphocyte line. The antigen-specific *in vitro* suppression was blocked by anti-CD8 antibody, demonstrating that suppression was dependent on CD8$^+$ T lymphocytes. As in EAE, EAU was also suppressed by feeding S-Ag related peptides that were either uveitogenic, cross reactive or synthetic (62-66). Gregerson et al., using high and low doses of S-Ag peptides, also found that low doses of antigen favor suppression whereas high doses induce unresponsiveness or anergy (65).

Diabetes. NOD diabetic mice spontaneously develop an autoimmune form of diabetes associated with insulitis. To test oral tolerance in the NOD model, we administered porcine insulin at a dose of 1 mg orally twice a week for five weeks and then weekly until one year of age (67). The severity of lymphocytic infiltration of pancreatic islets was reduced by oral administration of insulin, and there was a delay in the onset of diabetes. A decreased incidence of diabetes was seen in animals followed for one year. Suppression of insulitis as observed at a dose of 1 mg but not 5 mg. As expected, orally administered insulin had no metabolic affect on blood glucose levels. Furthermore, splenic T cells from animals orally treated with insulin adoptively transferred protection against diabetes, demonstrating that oral insulin generates active cellular mechanisms that suppress disease. Ongoing studies have demonstrated the ability to suppress insulitis by administering insulin peptides, the B chain of insulin, or GAD. Immunohistochemical studies have demonstrated an increase of IL-4 in the islets of insulin fed animals. Given the mechanism of antigen-driven bystander suppression, our results do not implicate autoreactivity to insulin as a pathogenic mechanism in the NOD mouse. Indeed, initial experiments suggest that orally administered glucagon can suppress insulitis.

TREATMENT OF AUTOIMMUNE DISEASES IN HUMANS

The first attempts of oral tolerization may have been utilized by Native Americans who were thought to have fed their children *Rhus* leaves to prevent them from becoming sensitized to poison ivy (68). Investigators have shown that exposure of a contact-sensitizing agent via the mucosa prior to subsequent skin challenge led to unresponsiveness in a portion of the subjects studied (69). In another study on human volunteers, serum antibodies to bovine serum albumin (BSA) were measured before and after feeding large amounts of this antigen (0.1 - 1.5 mg of BSA per pound per day). Those subjects that had anti-BSA antibodies prior to eating BSA showed a rise in their serum anti-BSA titers. A similar response was observed when some subjects were given an injection of BSA. Subjects who did not have anti-BSA antibodies before or after the test did not respond to subsequent intradermal immunization (70). Oral desensitization has also been attemped in Rh disease (71). In an attempt at oral immunization, human volunteers were given capsules containing killed streptococcus mutans and circulating IgA producing cells were found in some subjects (72). This suggests that some generation of a secretory immune response can occur following oral ingestion of microbial antigens. Orally administered KLH, 50 mg given daily for two weeks over a three week period, has been reported to decrease subsequent cell-mediated immune responses, although antibody responses were not affected (73). In addition, preliminary experiments in subjects fed KLH have suggested that cell lines may be generated that suppress proliferative responses although more work is needed in this area (74).

Multiple Sclerosis. In order to deterimine whether orally ingested autoantigens could affect the clinical course and immune responses in patients with an autoimmune disease, 15 patients with relapsing remitting multiple sclerosis were fed a capsule containing 300 mg of bovine myelin or placebo daily for one year (75). The results demonstrated a decrease in myelin basic protein reactive cells in the bloodstream of MS patients as compared to controls. There was no evidence of sensitization either as measured by antibody levels to MBP or PLP, or by increased proliferative responses to the fed antigens at a one year period. Clinical responses demonstrated that 12 of 15 placebo-fed patients had major MS attacks, whereas only 6 of 15 in the control group had attacks (p = 0.06). It appeared that a subgroup of patients that were either males or DR^{2-} preferentially responded to the oral tolerization. However the sample size was small and the degree to which this subgroup response will occur in future studies is unknown. Based on these observations, a multicenter 520 patient double-blind placebo controlled trial of bovine myelin in DR2- relapsing remitting MS patients, both males and females, has begun. Of note is that trials of myelin basic protein given by multiple subcutaneous injections resulted in prominent immune responses to the antigen (76).

Rheumatoid Arthritis. A 60-patient double-blind trial of oral collagen administration to patients with rheumatoid arthritis demonstrated a decrease in joint swelling and disease index in patients fed collagen compared to placebo controls (77) Patients were previously or currently on immunosuppressant drugs, such as methotrexate, that had failed such therapy. Patients were taken off these medications and treated for a 3 month period. In the first month, they received 100 mg of oral collagen per day, and in the second and third months 500 mg per day. These doses were extrapolated from the small amounts of collagen used to suppress adjuvant arthritis in the Lewis rat. There were no toxicities or evidence of sensitization to type II collagen in fed patients as measured by anticollagen antibodies. There was no linkage to either DR type or sex in the patients that responded. In patients treated with the collagen there was less need for narcotic use during the course of the study, and 4 patients in the collagen-treated group apparently had complete remission of their rheumatoid arthritis. Given the biologic effects seen, future trials will focus on other disease categories, more prolonged administration, and dosing studies. A multicenter trial is currently being planned. Given what is known of the mechanism of oral tolerization, these studies do not establish that type II collagen is a target autoantigen in the disease. Indeed, given the low doses fed, it is possible that the effect may have been mediated by regulatory cells that migrated to the joint and released anti-inflammatory cytokines such as TGFb or IL-4. Whether patients that went into complete remission represent a separate category remains to be determined.

Uveitis. An open-label pilot study has been performed on two patients with uveitis, one with Bechet's disease (78) and the second with pars planitis. In this open label trial, patients had required steroids and/or cyclosporin to maintain visual function. Patients were started on 30 mg of bovine S-antigen three times a week, and then tapered from steroids and immunosuppressive mediation. A positive therapeutic response was observed in both patients in that over a two year period they were able to reduce their previous medication without worsening of vision and with decrease in S-antigen responsiveness. A double-masked placebo-controled trial of 45 patients is currently in progress.

Future Directions. Given the results in animal models of autoimmunity and initial studies in human disease states, it appears that orally administered autoantigens may find a place for the treatment of human organ-specific inflammatory autoimmune diseases. Such therapy would have the advantages of being orally-administered, non-toxic, and antigen-specific. The mechansim of bystander suppression solves a major problem related to designing antigen or T cell specific therapy of inflammatory autoimmune diseases, since one need not necessarily identify the target autoantigen for oral tolerance to be effective. As discussed above, it is likely that in human autoimmune disease states, there are reactivities to multiple autoantigens from the target organ and multiple epitopes given that humans are an outbred population. Dosing appears to be important for stimulating the active suppression component of oral tolerance, and identification of regulatory cells in humans following oral tolerization is critical for demonstrating the immunologic effects of oral tolerization. Given the results in animal studies, one would predict that homologous protein and the use of synergist or enhancers would increase the biologic efficiency of oral tolerance. In this regard, recombinant human proteins and the concomitant administration of immune adjuvants to enhance generation of regulatory cells would be required.

REFERENCES

1. Harding CV, Unanue ER. Quantitation of antigen-presenting cell MHC class II/peptide complexes necessary for T-cell stimulation. Nature 1990; 346: 574-576.

2. Adorini L, Muller, S, Cardineaux F, Lehmann P, Falcioni F, Nagy ZA. In vivo competition between self peptides and foreign antigens in T-cell activation. Nature 1988; 334:623-625.

3. Woodroofe MN, Bellamy AS, Feldamnn M, Davison,AN, Cuzner ML. Immunocytochemical characterization of the immune reaction in the central nervous system in multiple sclerosis. Possible role for microglia in lesion growth. J Neurol Sci 1986; 74:135-152.

4. Hickey WF, Kimura HP. Perivascular microglial cells of the CNS are bone marrow-derived and present atigen in vivo. Science 1988; 239: 290-292.

5. Fontana A, Fierz W, Wekerle H. Astrocytes present myelin basic protein to encephalitogenic T-cell lines. Nature 1984; 307:273-276.

6. Fierz W, Endler B, Reske K, Wekerle HAF. Astrocytes as antigen-presenting cells. I. Induction of Ia antigen expression on astrocytes by T cells via immune interferon and its effect on atigen presentation. J Immunol 1985; 134:3785-3793.

7. Lisak RP, Zweiman B. In vitro cell-mediated immunity of cerebrospinal-fluid lymphocytes to myelin basic protein in primary demyelinating diseases. N Eng J Med 1977; 297:850-853.

8. Johnson D, Hafler DA, Fallis RJ, Lees MB, Brady RO, Quarles RH, Weiner HL. Cell-mediated immunity to myelin-associated glycoprotein, proteolipid protein, and myelin basic protein in multiple sclerosis. J Neuroimmunol 1986; 13:99-108.

9. Schluesener HJ, Wekerle H. Autoaggressive T lymphocyte lines recognozing the enecephaliogenic region of myelin basic protein: in vitro selection from unprimed rat T lymphocyte populations. J Immunol 1985; 135:3128-3133.

10. Martenson RE, Levine S, Sowinski R. The location of regions in guinea pig and bovine myelin basic proteins which induce experimental allergic encephalomyelitis in Lewis rats. J Immunol 1975; 114:592-595.

11. McFarlin DE, Blank SE, Kibler RF. Experimental allergic encephalomyelitis in the rat: response to encephalitogenic proteins and peptides. Science 1973; 179:478-480.

12. Vandenbark AA, Hashim GA, Celnik B. Determinants of human myelin basic protein that induce encephalitogenic T cells in Lewis rats. J Immunol 1989; 143:3512-3516.

13. Ota K, Matsui M, Milford EL, Mackin GA, Weiner HL, Hafler DA. T-cell recognition of immunodominant myelin basic protein epitope in multiple sclerosis. Nature 1990; 346:183-187.

14. Martin R, Howell MD, Jaraquemada D. A myelin basic protein peptide is recognized by cytotoxic T cells in th econtext of four HLA-DR types associated with multiple sclerosis. J Exp Med 1991; 173:19-24.

15. Jaraquemada D, Martin R, Rosen Bronson S, Flerlage M, McFarland H, Long EO. HLA-DR2a is the dominant restriction molecule for the cytotoxic T cell response to myelin basic protein in DR2Dw2 individuals. J Immunol 1990; 145:2880-2885.

16. Zhang JW, Chou CH, Hashim G, Medaer R, Raus JC. Preferential peptide specificity and HLA restriction of myelin basic protein-specific T cell clones derived from MS patients. Cell Immunol 1990; 129:189-198.

17. Wucherpfennig KW, Weiner HL, Hafler DA. T cell recognition of myelin basic protein. Immunol Today 1991; 12:277-282.

18. Chou YK, Vainiene M, Whitham R, Bourdette D, Chou CH, Hashim G, Offner H, Vandenbark AA. Response of human T lymphocyte lines to myelin basic protein: association of dominant epitopes with HLA class II restriction molecules. J Neurosci Res 1989; 23:207-216.

19. Pette M, Fujita K, Wilkinson D, Altmann DM, Trowsdale J, Giegrich G, Hinkkanen A, Epplen JT, Kappos L, Wekerle H. Myelin autoreactivity in multiple sclerosis: recognition of myelin basic protein in the context of HLA-DR2 products by T lymphocytes of multiple-sclerosis patients and healthy donors. Proc Natl Acad Sci USA 1990; 87:7968-7972.

20. Allegretta M, Nickals JA, Sriram S, Albertini RJ. T cells responsive to myelin basic protein in patients with multiple sclerosis. Science 1990; 247:718-721.

21. Kroemer G, Martinez AC. Mechanisms of cell tolerance. Immunol Today 1992; 13:401-404.

22. Miller JFAP, Moraham G. Peripheral T cell tolerance. Ann Rev Immunol 1992; 10:51-70.

23. Mowat AM. The regulation of immune reponses to dietary protein antigens. Immunol Today 1987; 8:93-98.

24. Whitacre CC, Gienapp IE, Orosz CG, Bitar D. Oral tolerance in experimental autoimmune encephalomyelitis. II. Evidence for clonal anergy. J Immunol 1991; 147:2155-2163.

25. Melamed D, Friedman A. Direct Evidence for anergy in T lymphocytes tolerized by oral administration of ovalbumin. Eur J Immunol 1993; 23:935-942.

26. Friedman A, Weiner Hl. Induction of anergy and/or active suppression in oral tolerance is determined by frequency of feeding and antigen dosage. FASEB Journal 1993; In Press

27. Miller A, Lider O, Roberts AB, Sporn MB, Weiner Hl. Suppressor T cells generated by oral tolerization to myelin basic protein suppresses both in vitro and in vivo immune responses by the release of TGF Beta following antigen specific triggering. Proc Natl Acad Sci USA 1992; 89:421-425.

28. Mowat AM, Strobel S, Drummond HE, Ferguson A. Immunological Response to fed protein antigens in mice: I. Reversal of oral tolerance to ovalbumin by cyclophosphamide. Immunology 1982; 45:105-113.

29. MacDonald TT. Immunosuppression caused by antigen feeding. I. Evidence for the activation of a feedback suppressor pathway in the spleens of antigen-fed mice. Eur J Immunol 1982; 12:767-773.

30. Guatam SC, Chikkala NF, Battisto JR. Oral administration of the contact sensitizer trinitrochlorobenzene: initial sensitization and subsequent appearance of a suppressor population. Cell Immunol 1990; 125:437-438.

31. Cowdery JS, Johlin BJ. Regulation of te primary in vitro response to TNP-polymerized ovalbumin by T suppressor cells induced by ovalbumin feeding. J Immunol 1984; 132:2783-2789.

32. Richman Lk, Chiller JM, Brown WR, Hanson DG, Vaz NM. Enterically induced immunological tolerance. I. Induction of suppressor T lymphocytes by intragastric administration of soluble proteins. J Immunol 1978; 121:2429-2433.

33. Strobel S, Mowat AM, Drummond HE, Pickering MG, Ferguson A. Immunological responses to fed protein antigen s in mice. II. Oral tolerance for CMI is due to activation of cyclophosphamide-sensitive cells by gut-processed antigen. Immunology 1983; 49:451-456.

34. Miller S, Hanson D. Inhibition of specific immune responses by feeding protein antigens. IV. Evidence for tolerance and specific active suppression of cell-mediated immune responses to ovalbumin. J Immunol 1979; 123:2344.

35. Bloom BR, Modlin RL, Salgame P. Stigma variations: observations on suppressor T cells and leprosy. Ann Rev Immunol 1992; 10:453-488.

36. Sercarz E, Krzych U. The distinctive specificity of antigen-specific suppressor T cells. Immunol Today 1991; 12:111-118.

37. Weiner Hl, Miller A, Khoury SJ, Al-SAbbagh A, Brod SA, Lider O, Higgins P, Sobel R, Matsui M, Sayegh M, Carpenter D, Eisnebarth G, Nussenblatt RB, Hafler DA. Suppression of organ-specific autoimmune diseases by oral administration of autoantigens. Progress in Immunol VIII: 8th Intl Congress of Immunol, Budapest 1992:627-634.

38. Lider O, Santos LMB, Lee CSY, Higgins PJ, Weiner HL. Suppression of experimental autoimmune encephalomyelitis by oral administration of myelin basic protein. II. Suppression of disease and in vitro immune reponses is mediated by antigen-specific CD8+ T lymphocytes. J Immunol 1989; 174:791-798.

39. Miller A, Prabhu-DAs M, Weiner HL. Epitopes of myelin basic protein (MBP) that trigger TGF Beta release following oral tolerization to MBP are different from encephalitogenic epitopes. FASEB Journal 1992; 6:1686.

40. Santos LMB, Al-Sabbagh A, Londono A, Weiner HL. Oral tolerance to myelin basic protein induces TGF Beta secreting T cells in Peyer's patches. J Immunol 1993; 150:115A.

41. Chen Y, Kuchroo V, Hafler DA, Weiner HL. Myelin basic protein specific regulatory T cell clones from orally tolerized mice suppress autoimmune encephalomyelitis. Science 1994; in press.

42. Schwartz RH. A cell culture model for T lymphocyte clonal anergy. Science 1990; 248:1349-1356.

43. DeSilva DR, Urdahl KB, Jenkins MK. Clonal anergy is induced in vitro by T cell receptor occupancy in the absence of proliferation. J Immunol 1991; 147:3261-3267.

44. Thompson HSG, Staines NA. Gastric administration of type II collagen delays the onset and severity of collagen-induced arthritis in rats. Clin Exp Immunol 1986; 64:581-586.

45. Nagler- Anderson C, Bober LA, Robinson ME, Siskind GW, Thorbeke FJ. Suppression of type II collagen -induced arthritis by intragastric administration of soluble type II collagen. Proc Natl Acad Sci USA 1986; 83:7443-7446.

46. Higgins PJ, Weiner HL. Suppression of experimental autoimmune encephalomyelitis by oral administration of myelin basic protein and its fragments. J Immunol 1988; 140: 440-445.

47. Brod SA, Al-Sabbagh A, Sobel RA, Hafler DA, Weiner HL. Suppression of experimental autoimmune encephalomyelitis by oral administration of myelin antigens. IV. Suppression of chronic relapsing disease in the Lewis rat and strain 13 guinea pig. Ann Neurol 1992; in press.

48. Miller A, Lider O, Al-Sabbagh A, Weiner HL. Suppression of experimental autoimmune encephalomyelitis by oral administration of myelin basic protein. V. Hierarchy of suppression by myelin basic protein from different species. J Neuroimmunol 1992; 39:243-250.

49. Bitar D, Whitacre CC. Suppression of experimental autoimmune encephalomyelitis by the oral administration of myelin basic protein. Cell Immunol 1988; 112:364-370.

50. Fuller KA, Pearl D, Whitacre CC. Oral tolerance in experimental autoimmune encephalomyelitis: Serum and salivary antibody responses. J Neuroimmunol 1990; 28:15-26.

51. Nussenblatt RB, CAspi RR, Mahdi R, Chan CC, Roberge F, Lider O, Weiner HL. Inhibition of S-antigen induced experimental autoimmune uveoretinitis by oral induction of tolerance with S-antigen. J Immunol 1990; 144:1689-1695.

52. Zhang JA, Davidson L, Eisenbarth G, Weiner HL. Suppression of diabetes in NOD mice by oral administration of porcine insulin. Proc Natl Acad Sci USA 1991; 88:10252-10256.

53. Bisaccia G, CAputo D, Landoni AM, MAcchi GP. Heterogeneity of human T lymphocytes to bind sheep red blood cells in multiple sclerosis patients and controls. Boll Inst Sieroter Milan 1978; 56:603-608.

54. Zhang JZ, Lee CSY, Lider O, Weiner HL. Suppression of adjuvant arthritis in Lewis rats by oral administration of type II collagen. J Immunol 1990; 145:2489-2493.

55. Birnbaum G, Lackovic V, Kotilinek L, Tobolt D. A comparison of regulatory cells in spinal fluid and blood in patients with multiple sclerosis and other neurologic diseases. Neurology 1990; 40:1785-1790.

56. Khoury SJ, Hancock WW, Weiner HL. Oral tolerance to myelin basic protein and natural recovery from experimental autoimmune encephalomyelitis are associated with down-regulation of inflammatory cytokines and differential upregulation of TGF Beta, IL-4 and PGE expression in the brain. J Exp Med 1992; 46:1355-1364.

57. Sayegh MH, Zhang ZJ, Hancock WW, Kwok CA, Carpenter Cb, Weiner HL. Down-regulation of the immune response to histocompatabilitys antigen and prevention of sensitization by skin allografts by orally administered alloantigen. Transplantation 1992; 53: 163-166.

58. Sayegh MH, Khoury SJ, Hancock WH, Weiner HL, Carpenter CB. Induction of immunity and oral tolerance with polymorphic class II major histocompatability complex allopeptides in the rat. Proc Natl Acad Sci USA 1992; 89:7762-7766.

59. Weiner HL, Friedman A, Miller A, Khoury SJ, Al-Sabbagh A, Santos L, Sayegh M, Nussenblatt RB, Trentham DE, Hafler DA. Oral tolerance: Immunologic mechanisms and treatment of animal and human organ specific autoimmune diseases by oral administration of autoantigens. Ann Rev Immunol 1994; in press.

60. Khoury SJ, Lider O, Al-Sabbagh A, Weiner HL. Suppression of experimental autoimmune encephalomyelitis by oral administration of myelin basic protein. III. Synergistic effect of lipopolysaccharide. Cell Immunol 1990; 88:404-407.

61. Thurau SR, Caspi RR, Chan CC, Weiner HL, Nussenblatt RB. Immunological suppression of experimental autoimmune uveitis. Fort Opthalmol 1991; 88:404-407.

62. Thurau SR, Chan CC, Suh E, Nussenblatt RB. Induction of oral tolerance to S-antigen induced experimental autoimmune uveitis by a uveitogenic 20mer peptide. J Autoimmunity 1991; 4:507-516.

63. Singh VK, Kalra HK, Yamaki K, Shinohara T. Suppression of experimental autoimmune uveitis in rats by the oral administration of the uveitopathogenic S-antigen fragment ar a cross-reactive homologous peptide. Cell Immunol 1992; 139:81-90.

64. Vrabec TR, Gregerson DS, Dua HS, Donoso LA. Inhibition of experimental autoimmune

uveoretinitis by oral administration of s-antigen and synthetic peptides. Autoimmunity 1992; 12:175-184.

65. Gregeerson D, Obritsch W, Donoso LA. Suppression of clonal anergy play roles in oral tolerance and EAU. Invest Opthalmol Vis Sci 1993; 34(suppl)(1000-5:45):902.

66. Suh EDW, Vistica B, Chan CC, Raber JM, Gery I, Nussenblatt RB. Splenectomy abrogatees the induction of oral tolerance in experimental autoimmune uveoretinitis. Current Eye Research in press.

67. Weiner HL, Zhang ZJ, Khoury SJ, Miller A, Al-Sabbagh A, Brod SA, Lider O, Higgins P, Sobel R, Nussenblatt RB, Hafler DA. Antigen-driven peripheral immune tolerance. Suppression of organ-specific autoimmune diseases by oral administration of autoantigens. Ann NY Acad Sci 1991; 636:227-232.

68. Dakin R. Remarks on a cutaneous affection produced by certain poisonous vegetables. Am J Med Sci 1829; 4:98-100.

69. Lowney ED. Immunologic unresponsiveness to a contact sensitizer in man. J Invest Dermatol 1968; 51:411-417.

70. Korenblatt PE, Rothberg RM, Minden P, Farr RS. Immune responses of human adults after oral and parenteral exposure to bovine serum albumin. J Allergy 1968; 41:226-235.

71. Gold WRJ, Queenan FT, Woody J, Sacher RA. Am J Obstet Gyecol 1983; 146:980.

72. Czerinsky C, Prince SJ, Michalek SM, Jackson S, Russell MW, Moldoveanu Z, McGhee JR, Mestecky J. IgA antibody-producing cells in peripheral blood after antigen ingeation: evidence for a common mucosal immune system in humans. Proc Natl Acad SCi USA 1987; 84:2449-2453.

73. Husby S, Elson CO, Moldoveanu Z, Mestecky J. Oral tolerance in humans. T cell but not B cell tolerance to a soluble protein antigen. 7th Intl Congress Mucosal Immunol 1992; Prague, Czechoslavakia.

74. Polanski M, Matsui M, Khoury S, Weiner HL. Oral tolerization to KLH in humans: generation of antigen-specific lines that suppress proliferative responses. J Immunol 1993; 150:114A.

75. Weiner HL, Mackin GA, Matsui M, Orav EJ, Khoury SJ, Dawson DM, Hafler DA. Double-blind pilot trial of oral tolerization with myelin antigens in multiple sclerosis. Science 1993; 259:1321-1324.

76. Salk RJS. A study of myelin basic protein as a therapeutic probe in patients with multiple sclerosis. Multiple Sclerosis 1983; Hallpike JK, Adams CWM, Toutellotte, editors.:Univerity Press, 1983:621-630.

77. Trentham DE, Dynesius-Trentham RA, Orav EJ, Combitchi D, Lorenzo C, Sewell KL, Hafler DA, WEiner HL. Effects of oral administration of type II collagen on rheumatoid arthritis. Science 1993; 261:1727-1730.

78. Nussenblatt RB, Smet D, Weiner HL, Grey I. The treatment of the ocular complications of Behcet's disease with oral tlerization. In: 6th Intl Conf on Behcet's Disease. 1993; Amsterdam(Elsevier Press, in press).

AAS 47
Inflammation:
Mechanisms and Therapeutics
© 1995 Birkhäuser Verlag Basel

CYTOPLASMIC TRANSCRIPTION FACTORS:
MEDIATORS OF CYTOKINE SIGNALING

D. E. Levy, R. Raz, J. E. Durbin, H. Bluyssen, R. Muzaffar, and S. Pisharody

Department of Pathology and Kaplan Comprehensive Cancer Center, NYU School of Medicine, 550 First Avenue, New York, NY 10016 USA

SUMMARY: The distinct pattern of transcriptional responses of cells to different extracellular signals requires a signal transduction pathway that provides rapid, accurate, and faithful transmission of information from the cell surface to the nucleus. One mechanism exploited by many cytokines, exemplified by interferons (IFN) but also used by many interleukins and growth factors, uses a family of cytoplasmic transcription factors that are activated by tyrosine phosphorylation. Once phosphorylated by receptor-associated tyrosine kinases, these proteins assemble into multimeric transcription factors, translocate to the nucleus, and bind specific DNA sequence elements in the promoters of target genes.

INTRODUCTION

The cellular response to cytokines, growth factors, and inflammatory mediators involves production of sets of specific proteins. Much of this response is the result of transcriptional induction of gene expression, with each distinct cytokine inducing a characteristic set of genes. The specificity of cytokine action is mediated by the distinct specificities of the cell surface receptor, each receptor binding and responding only to its cognate ligand. A conceptual problem toward understanding pathways propagating cytokine-activated transcriptional signals is the mechanism by which a ligand-occupied receptor delivers information accurately and faithfully to the nucleus. Cytokine receptors are transmembrane proteins consisting of extracellular domains involved in ligand recognition and binding, and cytoplasmic domains necessary for propagating signals. However, their cytoplasmic domains often have no recognizable enzymatic function. Rather, they appear to serve as links to cytoplasmic signaling systems. Experimental data on IFN-induced transcriptional responses have provided a paradigm applicable to a wide variety of cytokine and growth factor signaling that chart a pathway of receptor-activated signals from the cell surface to the nucleus (1).

IFN STIMULATED GENES

IFNs are antiviral and antiproliferative agents produced during the inflammatory response (2). They consist of two distantly-related families of cytokines, type I (IFNα/β) produced by leukocytes and fibroblasts and type II (IFNγ) produced by activated T lymphocytes. These two families of cytokines bind distinct cell surface receptors, activate different, though partially overlapping sets of genes, and produce distinctive cellular responses. Analysis of the mechanisms of transcriptional activation of IFNα stimulated genes provided details of the receptor-activated signaling pathway (3).

IFNα-stimulated genes contain a DNA enhancer element in their promoters that serves as the proximal target of the receptor-generated signal. This element, termed ISRE for IFNα stimulated response element, is necessary and sufficient for a transcriptional response to IFNα and is capable of transferring IFNα sensitivity to a reporter. In like manner, IFNγ -stimulated genes contain a distinct element in their promoters, termed GAS for gamma activated site, that renders them sensitive to the inducing effects of IFNγ (4). Thus, the specificity of signaling from these two receptor systems reduces to targeting through distinct DNA enhancer elements.

The ISRE of IFNα-stimulated genes binds a transcription factor detectable in the nucleus of IFNα treated cells. This transcription factor, termed ISGF3 for IFNα-stimulated gene factor, is composed of four distinct polypeptides (5, 6). These polypeptides are present in unstimulated cells; however, they fail to bind DNA prior to exposure of cells to IFNα. In fact, ISGF3 polypeptides are found in the cytoplasm of unstimulated cells rather than in the nucleus. Exposure of cells to IFNα causes these proteins to assemble into a multimeric complex and migrate to the nucleus (7, 8). In like manner, cells exposed to IFNγ display a DNA-binding activity targeted for the GAS element. This activity is composed of polypeptides sequestered in the cytoplasm of untreated cells that again assemble into a complex and migrate to the nucleus in response to IFNγ treatment (9).

TRANSCRIPTION FACTORS AS SIGNALING MOLECULES

Cytoplasmic transcription factors provide a direct link between activated cell surface receptors and the transcriptional induction of gene expression in response to IFN treatment. Purification of the protein components of ISGF3 and GAF and isolation of their corresponding cDNA clones has led to an elucidation of this signaling pathway. ISGF3 is composed of two dissociable subunits: one, termed ISGF3γ, is required for recognition of DNA while the second, termed ISGF3α, is the target for IFNα signaling. ISGF3γ is composed of a single, 48 kDa polypeptide that shares sequence homology with the interferon regulatory factor (IRF) family of transcription factors (10). This family of proteins contains an amino-terminal, DNA-binding domain displaying a tryptophan repeat reminiscent of the DNA-binding domain of the c-*myb* proto-oncoprotein and a carboxyl-terminal domain required for transcriptional activity. In the case of ISGF3γ p48, this carboxyl-terminal domain is required for interaction with the ISGF3α polypeptides during transcription factor assembly and nuclear translocation.

In addition, the carboxyl-terminal domain of ISGF3γ p48 plays a role in DNA recognition. The 48 kDa protein and carboxyl-terminal bind 11 bp of the ISRE. However, fully assembled ISGF3 recognizes a 13-14 bp segment of the ISRE, with the restriction in DNA recognition specificity deriving from one or more of the ISGF3α polypeptides in the complex (11). This ability of combinatorial association of proteins to produce distinct DNA binding specificities is key to propagation of multiple cytokine-derived signals using a limited number of signaling molecules. The ability of ISGF3α to alter the DNA-binding specificity of ISGF3γ p48 indicated that one or more of these proteins must directly interact with DNA. Indeed, when the protein composition was determined for GAF, the transcription factor activated by IFNγ, it was found to contain ISGF3 polypeptides. However, assembled in a different complex, they displayed a distinct DNA-binding target (12).

ISGF3α, the signaling target of the ISGF3 complex, is composed of three polypeptides of 84, 91, and 113 kDa. The 84 and 91 kDa proteins are shared with the GAF complex. These proteins are highly related: the 84 and 91 kDa proteins are derived from a single gene by alternative mRNA splicing, while the 113 kDa protein is derived from a separate gene showing approximately 35% amino acid identity (13, 14). These proteins share several conserved motifs: an amino-terminal basic domain thought to be involved in DNA recognition, a heptad repeat of hydrophobic amino acids that could form a coiled-coil interaction domain, and a Src-homology (SH) 2 domain that interacts with tyrosine phosphorylated peptides. In addition, there is sequence homology with SH3 domains and a conserved, carboxyl-terminal tyrosine. The conserved tyrosine has been found to become phosphorylated immediately following IFN treatment (15). This phosphorylation event is the primary switch for IFN signaling.·

THE PHOSPHORYLATION SWITCH

ISGF3 proteins in unstimulated cells are devoid of phosphotyrosine. Following exposure of cells to IFN, they become phosphorylated on a single tyrosine residue with the same kinetics as transcription factor assembly and gene activation. Tyrosine phosphorylation facilitates transcription factor assembly through SH2-phosphotyrosine mediated dimerization (16). The phosphotyrosine on one protein molecule is recognized by the SH2 domain of a second molecule while the SH2 domain of the first recognizes the phosphotyrosine of the second in reciprocal fashion. This forms a very stable, double dimerization interface. SH2-mediated dimerization may also stabilize additional interactions between heptad repeats, creating a structure resembling a leucine zipper model. Such a structure could place the amino-terminal basic regions in a conformation favorable for interaction with DNA.

Phosphorylation of ISGF3 proteins, like transcriptional induction, is a receptor-mediated event. Mouse cells are ordinarily insensitive to human IFN due to restricted receptor recognition. Transfection of mouse cells with an IFNα receptor component renders them sensitive to one species of human IFN, IFNαB. The cytoplasmic domain of this transmembrane protein, although not necessary for ligand recognition and displaying no obvious enzymatic function, is absolutely essential for ISGF3 activation in response to human IFNαB. Somatic cell genetic analysis of the human genes required to confer complete sensitivity for human IFNα/β on mouse cells implicated three distinct loci, all on human chromosome 21. Two of these genes have been cloned and encode members of the type II cytokine receptor family (17, 18).

The cytoplasmic domains of the IFNα receptor are necessary for ISGF3 tyrosine phosphorylation and activation. Since these receptors are not themselves tyrosine kinases, other enzymes must be involved in this response. It has been found that kinases of the Jak family are required for IFN signaling. The enzymes Tyk2 and Jak1 are required for IFNα signaling and Jak1 and Jak2 are required for IFNγ signaling (19-22). These enzymes are normally silent in cells; upon stimulation by IFN, they auto/trans-phosphorylate and acquire kinase activity toward exogenous substrates. Biochemical evidence suggests that the Jak kinases bind the cytoplasmic tails of receptors. Receptor aggregation following ligand binding probably facilitates kinase juxtaposition and cross phosphorylation. In many cases, the receptor itself also becomes tyrosine phosphorylated. Given the phosphotyrosine recognizing SH2 domains on ISGF3 proteins, such tyrosine phosphorylation would be essential for a likely model for receptor coupling. Aggregated receptors following ligand binding would activate and become phosphorylated by Jak family kinases. Tyrosine phosphorylation of receptors would serve as a target for the SH2 domains of cytoplasmic ISGF3 proteins, causing them to become membrane associated and bringing them in proximity to activated kinases. These same kinases could then phosphorylate the transcription factor subunits. Assuming that divalent homo- and hetero-dimerization of phosphorylated ISGF3 proteins is favored over the monovalent interaction with receptor, these phosphorylated proteins would dimerize and release from the receptor and thus be free to migrate to the nucleus. Nuclear translocation might be facilitated by uncovering of a nuclear translocation signal created by juxtaposition of the amino-terminal basic regions on two adjacent ISGF3 proteins. In such a model, the specificity inherent in ligand recognition of receptor would be faithfully translated into transcriptional activity through equally specific interactions between receptor tails and cytoplasmic transcription factors.

AN EXPANDING FAMILY OF TRANSCRIPTION FACTOR SIGNALING MOLECULES

The lessons learned from the IFN signaling pathway have led to elucidation of signaling pathways used by other cytokines. Indeed, some of the proteins discovered in the IFN pathway are shared by other cytokines. The 91 kDa ISGF3 protein essential for both IFNα and IFNγ signaling has been implicated in signaling from a variety of cell surface receptors (23). This protein becomes tyrosine phosphorylated in response to the growth factors EGF and PDGF, the lymphokines IL6, IL10, LIF, and OncoM, and the cytokine growth hormone. Additional members of the ISGF3 family have been discovered that become tyrosine phosphorylated in response to these and other cytokines, including IL2, IL3, IL4, erythropoietin, prolactin, and CSF1. This very general utilization of ISGF3-like transcription factors in signaling pathways has led to their designation as signal transducers and activators of transcription (STAT).

At present, at least six STAT proteins have been detected. STAT1 and 2 are the 91/84 and 113 kDa proteins of ISGF3; STAT3 is a protein 50% identical to STAT1 that is activated by IL6, among other cytokines, and constitutes the acute phase response factor (APRF) mediating activation of genes involved in the liver's acute phase response to inflammation. STAT4 is another related protein of as yet unknown function while STAT5 was characterized as a prolactin-responsive transcription factor in mammary gland. There is at least one, and most likely many, additional STAT proteins involved in responses to a variety of lymphokines and growth factors. The Jak kinases also represent an expanding family. Tyk2, Jak1, and Jak2 have been implicated in signaling not only from IFN receptors but also from erythropoietin, IL3, growth hormone, and the IL6 family of receptors. Recently, a fourth member of the Jak family, Jak3, was found associated with IL2 and IL4 receptors (24).

The Jak-STAT pathway is a flexible signaling system for coupling extracellular ligands to transcriptional responses. The multitude of STAT proteins, in conjunction with the Jak kinase family, provides an intracellular interface for cell surface receptors. Combinatorial assembly of multimeric transcription factors, composed of STAT proteins or STAT proteins in association with additional transcription factors such as members of the IRF family, modulates their DNA-binding specificities, targeting them to distinct DNA response elements to activate individual sets of genes.

ACKNOWLEDGEMENTS

R.R. is a fellow of the CSIC (Spain), J.E.D. is a postdoctoral fellow of the American Cancer Society, S.P. is a predoctoral fellow of the National Institutes of Health, and D.E.L. is a Pew Scholar. Work in the authors' laboratory was funded by grants from the National Institutes of Health and the Cancer Research Institute.

REFERENCES

1.   Levy DE, Darnell JE. Interferon-dependent transcriptional activation: signal transduction without second messenger involvement? New Biologist 1990; 2:923-928.

2.   De Maeyer E, De Maeyer-Guignard J. Interferons and other regulatory cytokines. New York: John Wiley & Sons, 1988: 1-448.

3.   Pellegrini S, Schindler C. Early events in signalling by interferons. Trends Biochem Sci 1993; 18:338-42.

4.   Lew DJ, Decker T, Strehlow I, Darnell JE. Overlapping elements in the guanylate-binding protein gene promoter mediate transcriptional induction by alpha and gamma interferons. Mol Cell Biol 1991; 11:182-191.

5.   Kessler DS, Veals SA, Fu XY, Levy DE. IFN-alpha regulates nuclear translocation and DNA-binding affinity of ISGF3, a multimeric transcriptional activator. Genes Dev 1990; 4:1753-1765.

6.   Fu XY, Kessler DS, Veals SA, Levy DE, Darnell JE. ISGF3, the transcriptional activator induced by interferon alpha, consists of multiple interacting polypeptide chains. Proc Natl Acad Sci USA 1990; 87:8555-8559.

7.   Levy DE, Kessler DS, Pine R, Darnell JE. Cytoplasmic activation of ISGF3, the positive regulator of interferon-alpha-stimulated transcription, reconstituted in vitro. Genes Dev 1989; 3:1362-1371.

8.   Dale TC, Imam A, Kerr IM, Stark GR. Rapid activation by interferon alpha of a latent DNA-binding protein present in the cytoplasm of untreated cells. Proc Natl Acad Sci USA 1989; 86:1203-1207.

9.   Decker T, Lew DJ, Mirkovitch J, Darnell JE. Cytoplasmic activation of GAF, an IFN-gamma-regulated DNA-binding factor. Embo J 1991; 10:927-932.

10.   Veals SA, Schindler C, Leonard D, Fu XY, Aebersold R, Darnell JE, Levy DE. Subunit of an alpha-interferon-responsive transcription factor is related to interferon regulatory factor and myb families of DNA-binding proteins. Mol Cell Biol 1992; 12:3315-3324.

11.   Veals SA, Santa Maria T, Levy DE. Two domains of ISGF3gamma that mediate protein-DNA and protein-protein interaction during transcription factor assembly contribute to DNA-binding specificity. Mol Cell Biol 1993; 13:196-206.

12.   Shuai K, Schindler C, Prezioso VR, Darnell JE. Activation of transcription by IFN-gamma: tyrosine phosphorylation of a 91-kD DNA binding protein. Science 1992; 258:1808-1812.

13.   Fu XY, Schindler C, Improta T, Aebersold RH, Darnell JE. The proteins of ISGF3, the IFN alpha-induced transcriptional activator, define a gene family involved in signal transduction. Proc Natl Acad Sci USA 1992; 89:7840-7843.

14.   Schindler C, Fu XY, Improta T, Aebersold RH, Darnell JE. Proteins of transcription factor ISGF3: one gene encodes the 91- and 84-kDa ISGF3 proteins that are activated by interferon alpha. Proc Natl Acad Sci USA 1992; 89:7836-7839.

15.   Schindler C, Shuai K, Prezioso VR, Darnell JE. Interferon-dependent tyrosine phosphorylation of a latent cytoplasmic transcription factor. Science 1992; 257:809-813.

16.   Shuai K, Horvath CM, Huang LHT, Qureshi SA, Cowburn D, Darnell JE. Interferon activation of the transcription factor Stat91 involves dimerization through SH2-phosphotyrosyl peptide interactions. Cell 1994; 76:821-828.

17.   Uzé G, Lutfalla G, Gresser I. Genetic transfer of a functional human interferon alpha receptor into mouse cells: Cloning and expression of its cDNA. Cell 1990; 60:225-234.

18.   Novick D, Cohen B, Rubinstein M. The human interferon alpha/beta receptor: characterization and molecular cloning. Cell 1994; 77:391-400.

19.   Velazquez L, Fellous M, Stark GR, Pellegrini S. A protein tyrosine kinase in the interferon alpha/beta signaling pathway. Cell 1992; 70:313-322.

20.   Müller M, Briscoe J, Laxton C, Buschlin D, Ziemiecki A, Silvennoinen O, Harpur AG, Barbieri G, Witthuhn BA, Schindler C, Pellegrini S, Wilks AF, Ihle JN, Stark GR, Kerr IM. The protein tyrosine kinase JAK1 complements defects in interferon-α/β and -γ signal transduction. Nature 1993; 366:129-135.

21.   Watling D, Guschin D, Müller M, Silvennoinen O, Witthuhn BA, Ihle JN, Stark GR, Kerr IM. Complementation of a mutant cell line defective in the interferon-gamma signal transduction pathway by the protein tyrosine kinase Jak2. Nature 1993; 366:166-170.

22.   Silvennoinen O, Ihle JN, Schlessinger J, Levy DE. Interferon-induced nuclear signaling by Jak protein tyrosine kinases. Nature 1993; 366:583-585.

23.   Darnell JE, Kerr IM, Stark GR. Jak-STAT pathways and transcriptional activation in response to IFNs and other extracellular signaling proteins. Science 1994; 264:1415-1420.

24.   Ihle JN. The Janus kinase family and signaling through members of the cytokine receptor superfamily. Proc Soc Exp Biol Med 1994; 206:268-272.

AAS 47
Inflammation:
Mechanisms and Therapeutics
© 1995 Birkhäuser Verlag Basel

PROTEIN KINASE C IN CELL SIGNALING: STRATEGIES FOR THE DEVELOPMENT OF SELECTIVE INHIBITORS

P.M. Blumberg, G. Acs, P. Acs, L.B. Areces, M.G. Kazanietz, N.E. Lewin, and Z. Szallasi

Molecular Mechanisms of Tumor Promotion Section, Laboratory of Cellular Carcinogenesis and Tumor Promotion, National Cancer Institute, Bethesda, MD 20892-4255, U.S.A.

SUMMARY: Protein kinase C plays a central role in the cellular signaling pathway for the lipophilic second messenger sn-1,2-diacylglycerol, which is involved in many biological responses, including tumor promotion and inflammation. A major effort has been directed at understanding diversity within this system in order to develop strategies for selective inhibition. Two classes of ligands for the regulatory domain of protein kinase C have been identified which, although they function in vitro as activators of the enzyme, paradoxically behave in vivo as partial antagonists. Identification of targets for the phorbol esters distinct from protein kinase C argues that antagonists acting on the regulatory and catalytic domains of protein kinase C will have different spectra of action.

Croton oil, the seed oil of Croton tiglium, was prominent in the pharmacopoeia of earlier times as a counter-irritant and cathartic. Efforts to define the role of inflammation in carcinogenesis led to the characterization of croton oil as the paradigm for a class of cancer causing agents called **tumor promoters**. Based on short-term assays for inflammation, the active constituents from croton oil were identified to be a series of diesters of the tetracyclic diterpene phorbol, and numerous derivatives were subsequently found in plants of the family Euphorbiaceae (1). Biologically, the phorbol esters induced an impressive array of responses, suggesting that they were functioning in some central pathway of cellular control (2). Some years ago, this laboratory was able to demonstrate the existence of specific, high affinity receptors for the phorbol esters (3). The emerging similarities between these phorbol ester receptors and the enzyme protein kinase C suggested that these were different activities of the same protein (4). Indeed, the phorbol esters proved to activate protein kinase C, and phorbol ester binding activity copurified with the enzyme.

Over the past decade, much has been learned about the structure and function of protein kinase C. Protein kinase C is thought to mediate responses to the lipophilic second messenger sn-1,2-diacylglycerol, with the phorbol esters acting as ultrapotent analogs of diacylglycerol (5). One prominent source of diacylglycerol during signaling is hydrolysis by phospholipase C of the lipid phosphatidylinositol-4,5-bisphosphate, generating not only diacyglycerol but also inositol-1,4,5-triphosphate, which in turn is coupled to elevation of intracellular calcium, an additional second messenger. It is now appreciated, however, that other routes for generation of diacylglycerol during cellular signaling also exist, such as indirect formation via phosphatidic acid produced by phospholipase D from phosphatidylcholine. In addition, other lipids produced during signaling, e.g. arachidonic acid or lysophosphatidylcholine, may play a synergistic role in the stimulation of protein kinase C (6).

Just as the simplistic early concepts regarding the production of diacylglycerol have ceded to recognition of temporally complex production of variable mixtures of lipophilic second messengers and comessengers, so protein kinase C has evolved from a single calcium and lipid dependent protein kinase to a growing family of related isozymes as revealed by cloning (7). In all cases, the isozymes consist of an N-terminal regulatory domain and a C-terminal catalytic domain. The catalytic domain acts as a serine/threonine specific protein kinase. The regulatory domain is thought to inhibit this catalytic activity through a so-called pseudosubstrate region near its N-terminus. Adjacent to this pseudosubstrate region is a pair of highly conserved zinc finger structures, which represent the phorbol ester binding domain on the molecule and which contribute to the requirement for anionic phospholipid. In the "classic" isozymes alpha, beta, and gamma, there is also a further domain (the C2 region) which is thought to confer the dependence on calcium. The "novel" isozymes delta, epsilon, eta, and theta lack this C2 region and correspondingly lack calcium dependence. The "atypical" isozymes zeta and iota both lack this C2 domain and possess only a single, somewhat divergent zinc finger region which is incapable of binding phorbol ester. The physiological mode of regulation of the "atypical" protein kinase C isozymes remains to be defined.

Within the cell, protein kinase C exists in both the soluble and particulate fractions, in proportions depending on the specific isozyme. Addition of phorbol ester has two effects. First, it causes the translocation of protein kinase C to the membrane fraction, concomitant with the activation of the enzyme. Second, by labilizing the activated protein kinase C to proteolysis the phorbol ester potentially leads to the longterm down-regulation of the enzyme, thereby terminating the activation.

The early analysis of phorbol ester structure activity relations clearly revealed that not all phorbol esters induced the same pattern of response (8). A major focus of our research effort has been to understand the biochemical basis for this heterogeneity. Such insight is necessary if we wish to predict the consequences of modifications in second messenger levels resulting from changes in oncogenes, growth factors, or the exposure to xenobiotics. Furthermore, the central role of protein kinase C in signal transduction suggests that it should be a promising therapeutic target. However, the success in exploiting this target for drug development will depend in part in strategies for endowing specificity for the response of interest.

One important basis for possible selectivity is the diversity among isozymes of protein kinase C. As summarized in Table 1, the isozymes can fulfill overlapping but distinct functions. Coupled

Table 1. Protein kinase C isozyme diversity

EFFECT	Cell Line	PKC α	PKC β	PKC δ	PKCε	Ref
Antigen induced secretion	RBL-2H3	+	+++	++	-	9
Inhibition of phospholipase C	RBL-2H3	+++	+	+	+++	9
c-fos/c-jun expression	RBL-2H3	-	+++	-	+++	10
Phosphorylation of the gamma chain of the IgE receptor	RBL-2H3	-	-	+++	-	11
Myeloid differentiation	32D	+++	-	+++	-	12
Cell growth	NIH 3T3	N.D.	N.D.	---	+++	13
Tumorigenicity in nude mice	NIH 3T3	N.D.	N.D.	-	+++	13

with different isozyme profiles in different cells, such functional differences between isozymes provide the strong prediction that different responses will be found in different cells.

A separate issue is how different ligands can produce different biological effects. Comparison of structure activity relations for binding of phorbol esters to protein kinase C isozymes in vitro reveals two patterns of selectivity (14). For some derivatives, such as the indole alkaloids or diacylglycerol, little selectivity is observed. For others, such as phorbol 12,13-dibutyrate, in vitro binding is somewhat weaker to the "novel" isozymes delta, epsilon, and eta than it is to the "classical" isozymes alpha, beta, and gamma. Binding characteristics are not only determined by the specific isozyme, however. We have observed dramatic differences in relative selectivity depending on the specific lipid environment in which the isozymes are reconstituted for the in vitro assays (15). For example, the bryostatin derivative Δ-19,20-isobryostatin 10 showed little selectivity between protein kinase C alpha and gamma in the presence of phosphatidylserine, whereas it showed markedly weaker affinity for protein kinase C gamma in the presence of a Triton X-100/phosphatidylserine mixture. In the intact cell, moreover, the selectivity of ligands for specific isozymes depends on the cell type examined. Thus, phorbol 12-myristate 13-acetate shows markedly higher selectivity for protein kinase C delta versus alpha in mouse keratinocytes than in NIH 3T3 cells (16, 17). We conclude that the in vitro assays are an unreliable measure of isozyme selectivity in the intact cell. As currently constituted, they are thus of limited value for drug development. A further implication is that the characteristics of protein kinase C are highly context dependent.

Differences in isozyme recognition, whether reflecting the structures of the isozymes per se or of their environment and modifications within the cell, predict possible differences in the pattern of response to various ligands. One of the surprises in the field, however, was that the diversity of observed response extended far beyond this. Two classes of ligands for protein kinase C have been identified which, although they activate protein kinase C in vitro, function in the intact cell as partial antagonists. These classes, exemplified by bryostatin 1 and by the 12-deoxyphorbol 13-monoesters prostratin and 12-deoxyphorbol 13-phenylacetate, prove the feasibility of partial agonists targeted to the regulatory domain of protein kinase C. Understanding the basis for their antagonistic action may permit the development of additional classes with different patterns of antagonism.

The conventional strategy for antagonizing protein kinase C has been through inhibition of the catalytic domain. This approach has received considerable attention by the pharmaceutical industry, and high affinity inhibitors with substantial selectivity vis-a-vis other kinases and some even with selectivity between the classic and novel protein kinase C isozymes have been obtained. Of great importance, initial reports suggest that such inhibitors may have limited toxicity, further supporting the attractiveness of protein kinase C as a therapeutic target. A conceptual difficulty with inhibitors of the catalytic domain of protein kinase C, however, is the relatively high level of similarity between all serine/threonine kinases and the large number of such kinases. Since in vitro evaluation can only assess selectivity for a limited panel of kinases, the observed in vitro selectivity will obviously be better than that which will actually occur in vivo.

The bryostatins were the first of the two classes of partial antagonists of protein kinase C acting through the regulatory domain. Derived from the marine bryozoan Bugula neritina, bryostatin 1 was isolated by Dr. George R. Pettit on the basis of its ability to extend the lifespan of mice inoculated with P388 tumor cells (18). Extensive characterization by my group and others has shown that bryostatin 1 induces in cell systems à subset of the responses observed for the typical phorbol esters; in virtually every instance in which bryostatin 1 fails to induce a typical phorbol ester response, bryostatin 1 blocks the response of the cells to the phorbol esters if both agents are applied together (19). Of particular importance, the bryostatins are inactive as complete or first stage tumor promoters in the mouse skin model and show only weak second stage tumor promoting activity (20). Bryostatin 1 is currently undergoing clinical trial in England.

Efforts to understand the mechanism for the unique pattern of activity of the bryostatins reveal both similarities and differences with the phorbol esters. The bryostatins activate in vitro all the protein kinase C isozymes examined to a similar extent as do the phorbol esters (15). In in vitro binding assays, moreover, they do not appear to display unusual isozyme selectivity. A number of striking differences have emerged, however. First, the bryostatins bind to protein kinase C with greatly enhanced affinity compared to the phorbol esters (21). Indeed, this high affinity complicates determination of equilibrium dissociation constants. An important implication of this high affinity is that the bryostatins at nM concentrations are present at concentrations orders of magnitude above their dissociation constant for protein kinase C; the bryostatins may therefore also interact with (relatively) low affinity receptors distinct from the usual phorbol ester targets. Consistent with this model, several of the unusual responses to the bryostatins can be mimicked by the phorbol esters at μM concentrations. Likewise, the antagonism of the phorbol ester responses by the bryostatins is non-competitive with the phorbol esters, consistent with its being mediated by a site to which the phorbol esters at typical concentrations fail to bind (16, 17). Such low affinity targets for the bryostatins could represent novel receptors; alternatively, they could reflect protein kinase C which is associated with cellular environments which fail to reconstitute the binding affinity properly.

A second difference between the bryostatins and the phorbol esters is that the bryostatins dissociate from protein kinase C with much slower kinetics than do the phorbol esters (22). In contrast to a dissociation rate at 37 °C of seconds to minutes for the phorbol esters, bryostatin 1 dissociates with a half-life of several hours. This time is similar to the half-life of protein kinase C in the cell in the presence of the bryostatin. We therefore predict that bryostatin could anchor protein kinase C at the first location within the cell at which it binds the bryostatin, preventing subsequent redistribution. Since protein kinase C can only phosphorylate substrates in proximity to the activated enzyme, differences in location of activated enzyme should translate into differences in substrate specificity. Consistent with this prediction, bryostatin but not phorbol ester was reported to induce localization of protein kinase C to the nuclear envelope and to cause the phosphorylation of lamin B (23).

The bryostatins not only show slower release from protein kinase C after binding but also show slower kinetics for inducing translocation of protein kinase C to the membrane (17). Whereas phorbol 12-myristate 13-acetate has similar ED_{50} values for translocation of protein kinase C alpha and epsilon at 5 min and 6 hours, bryostatin appears much more potent at the later time. Since protein kinase C isozymes can fulfill different functions within the cell, the first isozyme to be activated might block response to a subsequently activated isozyme.

In contrast to the in vitro binding assays, in intact 3T3 cells (16) and keratinocytes (17) the bryostatins show marked selectivity for the novel protein kinase C isozymes delta and epsilon compared to alpha. In addition, bryostatin 1 at high concentrations protects protein kinase C delta from down regulation either by itself or by phorbol ester. This protection is non-competitive, and the dose response curves for protection of protein kinase C delta correlate with the antagonism of phorbol ester effects on cJUN protein in 3T3 cells or on epidermal growth factor binding or cornification in mouse keratinocytes. The antagonism could reflect a critical role for protein kinase C delta in these processes. Alternatively, protection of protein kinase C delta may simply reflect the antagonism resulting from the action of bryostatin on some other target within the cell.

The second class of partial antagonists of protein kinase C acting through its regulatory domain is that of the 12-deoxyphorbol 13-monoesters, for which the best studied examples are prostratin (12-deoxyphorbol 13-acetate) and 12-deoxyphorbol 13-phenylacetate. Prostratin initially attracted interest when it was detected in a screen of plant extracts with anti-HIV activity (24). Initial characterization suggested that prostratin functioned as a typical phorbol ester in C3H10T1/2 fibroblasts with 20 or 40 fold weaker potency than phorbol 12,13-dibutyrate. Likewise, in in vitro binding assays prostratin showed typical selectivity for PKC isozymes, being modestly more potent for the classical isozymes, and it fully stimulated kinase activity (14).

In mouse skin, in contrast, prostratin induced relative to typical phorbol esters a weak response for some biological endpoints such as induction of ornithine decarboxylase, edema, or infiltration of neutrophils. For other responses, such as induction of hyperplasia or keratin K6, prostratin was entirely without activity. By analogy with bryostatin, for which antagonism of phorbol ester response was observed for all those responses that bryostatin itself failed to induce, we predicted that prostratin might likewise block induction of these responses by phorbol ester. This indeed proved to be the case. Prostratin pretreatment inhibited ornithine decarboxylase induction, edema, and infiltration of neutrophils by approximately 70%, and it completely prevented either acute or chronic hyperplasia (25, 26). This latter finding was of particular significance, since induction of chronic hyperplasia represents one of the best correlates with tumor promoting activity in skin. In fact, prostratin was able to inhibit papilloma formation by 97% (27). Prostratin thus affords a dramatic example of a protein kinase C activator which functions as an antitumor promoter. 12-deoxyphorbol 13-phenylacetate proved to behave in a generally similar fashion to prostratin, but with higher potency. The ED_{50} for inhibition of promotion by 12-deoxyphorbol 13-phenylacetate was 0.8 nmol per application. This derivative is thus more potent as an inhibitor of tumor promotion than is the most potent of the typical phorbol esters, phorbol 12-myristate 13-acetate, as a tumor promoter.

Like the bryostatins, the 12-deoxyphorbol 13-monoesters differ from typical phorbol esters in their kinetics and pattern of down regulation of protein kinase C isozymes in vivo (manuscript submitted). First, the 12-deoxyphorbol 13-monoesters cause the rapid translocation of all three isozymes alpha, delta, and epsilon in mouse keratinocytes. In contrast, bryostatin causes the slow translocation of all three isozymes and phorbol 12-myristate 13-acetate causes the slow translocation of protein kinase C delta. Second, in keratinocytes 12-deoxyphorbol 13-phenylacetate shows marked selectivity for the novel isozymes delta and epsilon compared to alpha. This in vivo selectivity is in dramatic contrast to the slightly higher potency for alpha than for the novel isozymes as indicated by the in vitro binding assays. Finally, in keratinocytes 12-deoxyphorbol 13-phenylacetate causes the complete down regulation of protein kinase C epsilon, in contrast to both phorbol 12-myristate 13-acetate and bryostatin, which cause down regulation of protein kinase C epsilon only from the cytosol and not from the particulate fraction. It is perhaps noteworthy that protein kinase C epsilon is unique among protein kinase C isozymes in its ability to transform fibroblasts upon overexpression.

As with binding affinity, the ability to down regulate protein kinase C is dependent on the cellular context. Whereas protein kinase C epsilon is fully down regulated by 12-deoxyphorbol 13-phenylacetate but not by bryostatin or phorbol 12-myristate 13-acetate in keratinocytes, in NIH 3T3 cells epsilon is fully down regulated by all three ligands, and in RBL-2H3 cells it is fully down regulated by none of the three ligands.

Conceptually, the identification of multiple isozymes of protein kinase C provided a facile explanation for the heterogeneity of response to the phorbol esters, a phenomenon which at the whole animal level had been unambiguously documented by Hecker and coworkers long before the discovery of protein kinase C (8). The recent identification of novel classes of high affinity receptors for the phorbol esters distinct from protein kinase C argues that the overall role of protein kinase C in phorbol ester action requires urgent reevaluation.

Two classes of novel receptors for the phorbol esters have been identified so far. The chimaerin class consists to four members. They contain an N-terminal zinc finger phorbol ester binding domain homologous to that in protein kinase C coupled to a C-terminal GTPase activation domain homologous to that in the breakpoint cluster region protein (28). This GTPase activating domain is recognized by p21rac. Although the full range of functions of p21rac remains to be defined, p21rac forms a component of the NADPH oxidase complex in neutrophils and is involved in membrane ruffling. In addition, p21rac controls the activity of p65[PAK], an upstream effector of the MAP kinase pathway. All these pathways are activated by phorbol ester. The involvement of chimaerin in phorbol ester action in most systems remains uncertain, however, because the currently identified members of the class are only found in brain and testes.

The second class of novel high affinity receptors for the phorbol esters is represented by a single member, so far identified only in the nematode Caenorhabditis elegans, and referred to as unc-13 (29). Unc-13 contains domains homologous to the C1 and C2 conserved regions of protein kinase C. As discussed previously, the C1 domain contains the phorbol ester binding zinc fingers, and the C2 domain confers the calcium dependence in the classical protein kinase C isozymes. The function of the effector domain of unc-13 remains to be determined, as does the possible presence of an unc-13 homolog in mammalian cells. Interestingly, the designation unc-13 refers to a gene which yields a uncoordinated phenotype upon mutation. In the nematode, one of the phenotypic effects of phorbol ester treatment is uncoordination (30).

We have compared n-chimaerin and protein kinase C alpha with respect to phorbol ester binding, phospholipid dependence, and sensitivity to inhibitors (31). Examining phorbol esters and related ligands chosen to represent the range of variation in biological response and spanning over three orders of magnitude in binding affinity, we observed no more than a 2-fold difference in binding to these two distinct phorbol ester receptors. In fact, n-chimaerin more closely resembles protein kinase C alpha in its binding characteristics than does protein kinase C epsilon. We similarly found close resemblance in the ED_{50} values for reconstitution of binding by phosphatidylserine and in the ability of different phospholipids to reconstitute binding. Finally, two "specific inhibitors" of protein kinase C which act upon the regulatory domain, viz. calphostin C and sphingosine, inhibited phorbol ester binding to n-chimaerin and protein kinase C alpha with indistinguishable potencies.

Comparison of the zinc finger domains of unc-13 and protein kinase C delta yielded generally similar conclusions (manuscript submitted). Absolute binding affinities for phorbol esters and related ligands were approximately the same, albeit 2-5 fold weaker for unc-13, and calphostin C inhibited both with similar potencies. Modest differences were observed in lipid requirements.

Both the chimaerin and unc-13 classes of phorbol ester receptors were identified from clones isolated for other purposes which upon sequencing proved to have homology to the zinc finger region of protein kinase C. It seems entirely plausible that a systematic search will reveal further distinct classes of phorbol ester receptors.

The close similarity in the properties of protein kinase C, the chimaerins, and unc-13 has several very important implications. First, the novel receptors and protein kinase C recognize diacylglycerol with similar affinities. The novel receptors therefore provide alternative pathways for signal transduction in response to diacylglycerol. The possible role of co-regulators of protein kinase C for discrimination between these multiple pathways now becomes an issue of great importance. Second, the binding of phorbol ester to these novel receptors, their similar structure-activity requirements, and their sensitivity to "specific protein kinase C inhibitors" which function through the regulatory domain mean that many of the tools that have been routinely used to implicate protein kinase C in a specific biological response are misleading, since they fail to distinguish between distinct receptor classes. Reevaluation of the role of protein kinase C in such biological responses through other experimental approaches, such as overexpression of specfic isozymes, use of dominant negative mutants, or antisense, is imperative. Third, efforts to antagonize protein kinase C have been directed at both the regulatory or catalytic domains of the molecule. These domains are shared by different subsets of effectors. The phorbol ester binding domain is present on unc-13, on the chimaerins, and on the classical and novel subclasses of protein kinase C. The catalytic domain of protein kinase C is found on the atypical subclass of protein kinase C as well as on the other subclasses, and considerable homology exists with other kinases. Obviously, the secondary targets affected by inhibitors directed at the catalytic and regulatory domains will therefore differ. The two approaches to inhibitor design should therefore be complementary.

A major theoretical concern in the development of inhibitors of protein kinase C has been the ability to separate therapeutic actions from undesired side effects arising from actions on protein kinase C in other systems. The multiplicity of isoforms of protein kinase C greatly enhances the opportunities for selectivity. Our findings indicate, furthermore, that the specific cellular environment in which protein kinase C is located makes a very marked contribution to its characteristics. The structure activity relations differed by orders of magnitude between in vitro and in vivo assays. Likewise, susceptibility to down regulation was a function of the specific cell type. Identification of the specific modifying factors in the cellular environment is a pressing objective. In any case, their existence provides great potential for obtaining diversity of response. Our experience with the limited compounds currently available provides strong encouragement that inhibitors of protein kinase C can afford useful therapeutic agents. Prostratin caused dramatic inhibition of tumor promotion in mice at tolerated doses (27); the catalytic site directed protein kinase C inhibitor Ro 32-0432 was orally tolerated in rats and inhibited adjuvant induced arthritis (32). The combination of medicinal chemistry and expanding mechanistic knowledge holds promise of further rapid progress.

REFERENCES

1. Hecker E. Structure-activity relationships in diterpene esters irritant and cocarcinogenic to mouse skin. In: Carcinogenesis, Vol. 2. Mechanisms of Tumor Promotion and Cocarcinogenesis. Slaga TJ, Sivak A, Boutwell RK, editors. New York: Raven Press, 1978: 11-48.

2. Blumberg PM. In vitro studies on the mode of action of the phorbol esters, potent tumor promoters. CRC Crit Rev Toxicol 1980; 8:153-234.

3. Driedger PE, Blumberg PM. Specific binding of phorbol ester tumor promoters. Proc Natl Acad Sci USA 1980; 77:567-571.

4. Blumberg PM. Protein kinase C as the receptor for the phorbol ester tumor promoters. Sixth Rhoads Memorial Award Lecture. Cancer Res 1988; 48:1-8.

5. Nishizuka Y. The role of protein kinase C in cell surface signal transduction and tumour promotion. Nature 1984; 308:693-698.

6.   Nishizuka Y. Intracellular signaling by hydrolysis of phospholipids and activation of protein kinase C. Science 1992; 258:607-614.

7.   Nishizuka Y. The molecular heterogeneity of protein kinase C and its implications for cellular regulation. Nature 1988; 334:661-665.

8.   Fürstenberger G, Hecker E. Zum Wirkungsmechanismus cocarcinogener Pflanzeninhaltsstoffe. Planta Medica 1972; 22:241-266.

9.   Ozawa K, Szallasi Z, Kazanietz MG, Blumberg PM, Mischak H, Mushinski JF, Beaven MA. Ca^{++}-dependent and Ca^{++}-independent isozymes of protein kinase C mediate exocytosis in antigen-stimulated rat basophilic RBL-2H3 cells: reconstitution of secretory responses with Ca^{++} and purified isozymes in washed permeabilized cells. J Biol Chem 1993; 268:1749-1756.

10. Razin E, Szallasi Z, Kazanietz MG, Blumberg PM, Rivera J. Protein kinase C-β and ε link the mast cell high affinity receptor for IgE to the expression of C-fos and c-jun. Proc Natl Acad Sci USA 1994; 91:7722-7726.

11. Germano P, Gomez J, Kazanietz MG, Blumberg PM, Rivera J. Phosphorylation of the γ chain of the high affinity receptor for immunoglobulin E by receptor-associated protein kinase C-δ. J Biol Chem 1994; 269:23102-23107.

12. Mischak H, Pierce JH, Goodnight J, Kazanietz MG, Blumberg PM, Mushinski JF. Phorbol ester-induced myeloid differentiation is mediated by protein kinase C-α and -δ and not by protein kinase C-βII, -ε, -zeta and eta. J Biol Chem 1993; 268:20110-20115.

13. Mischak H, Goodnight J, Kolch W, Martiny-Baron G, Schaechtle C, Kazanietz MG, Blumberg PM, Pierce JH, Mushinski JF. Overexpression of protein kinase C-δ and -ε in NIH 3T3 cells induces opposite effects of growth, morphology, anchorage dependence, and tumorigenicity. J Biol Chem 1993; 268:6090-6096.

14. Kazanietz MG, Areces LB, Bahador A, Mischak H, Goodnight J, Mushinski JF, Blumberg PM. Characterization of ligand and substrate specificity for the calcium-dependent and calcium-independent PKC isozymes. Mol Pharmacol 1993; 44:298-307.

15. Kazanietz MG, Lewin NE, Gao F, Pettit GR, Blumberg PM. Binding of [26-^{3}H]bryostatin 1 and analogs to calcium-dependent and calcium-independent PKC isozymes. Mol Pharmacol 1994; 46:374-379.

16. Szallasi Z, Smith CB, Pettit GR, Blumberg PM. Differential regulation of protein kinase C isozymes by bryostatin 1 and phorbol 12-myristate 13-acetate in NIH 3T3 fibroblasts. J Biol Chem 1994; 269:2118-2124.

17. Szallasi Z, Denning MF, Smith CB, Dlugosz AA, Yuspa SH, Pettit GR, Blumberg PM. Bryostatin 1 protects PKCδ from down-regulation in mouse keratinocytes in parallel with its inhibition of phorbol ester induced differentiation. Mol Pharmacol 1994; (in press)

18. Pettit GR, The bryostatins. Prog Chem Org Nat Prod 1991; 57:153-212.

19. Blumberg PM, Pettit GR. The bryostatins, a family of protein kinase C activators with therapeutic potential. In: Krogsgaard-Larsen P, Christensen SB, Kofod H, eds. New Leads and Targets in Drug Research, Alfred Benzon Symposium 33. Copenhagen: Munksgaard International, 1992:273-285.

20. Hennings H, Blumberg PM, Pettit GR, Herald CL, Shores R, Yuspa SH. Bryostatin 1, an activator of protein kinase C, inhibits tumor promotion by phorbol esters in SENCAR mouse skin. Carcinogenesis 1987; 8:1343-1346.

21. deVries DJ, Herald CL, Pettit GR, Blumberg PM. Demonstration of subnanomolar affinity of bryostatin 1 for the phorbol ester receptor in rat brain. Biochem Pharmacol 1988; 37:4069-4073.

22. Lewin NE, Dell'Aquila ML, Pettit GR, Blumberg PM, Warren BS. Binding of ^{3}H-Bryostatin 4 to protein kinase C. Biochem.Pharmacol. 1992; 43:2007-2014.

23. Fields AP, Pettit GR, May WS. Phosphorylation of lamin B at the nuclear membrane by activated protein kinase C. J Biol Chem 1988; 263:8253-8260.

24. Gustafson KR, Cardellina II JH Jr, McMahon JB, Gulakowski RT, Ishitoya JI, Szallasi Z, Lewin NE, Blumberg PM, Weislow OS, Beutler JA, Cox PA, Buckheit RW, Cragg GM, Bader JP, Boyd MR. A nonpromoting phorbol from the samoan medicinal plant Homalanthus nutans inhibits cell killing by HIV-1. J Med Chem 1992; 35:1978-1986.

25. Szallasi Z, Blumberg PM. Prostratin, a non-promoting phorbol ester, inhibits induction by phorbol 12-myristate 13-acetate of ornithine decarboxylase, edema, and hyperplasia in CD-1 mouse skin. Cancer Res 1991; 51:5355-5360.

26. Szallasi Z, Krausz KW, Blumberg PM. Non-promoting 12-deoxyphorbol 13-esters as potent inhibitors of phorbol 12-myristate 13-acetate induced acute and chronic biological responses. Carcinogenesis 1992; 13:2161-2167.

27. Szallasi Z, Krsmanovic L, Blumberg PM. Non-promoting 12-deoxyphorbol 13-esters inhibit phorbol 12-myristate 13-acetate induced tumor promotion in CD-1 mouse skin. Cancer Res 1993; 53:2507-2512.

28. Lim L. N-chimaerin and neuronal signal transduction mechanisms. Biochem Soc Trans 1992; 20:611-614

29. Ahmed S, Maruyama IN, Kozma R, Lee J, Brenner S, Lim L. The Caenorhabditis elegans unc-13 gene product is a phospholipid-dependent high affinity phorbol ester receptor. Biochem J 1992; 287:995-999.

30. Lew KK, Chritton S, Blumberg PM. Biological responsiveness to the phorbol esters and specific binding of [^{3}H]phorbol 12,13-dibutyrate in the nematode Caenorhabditis elegans, a manipulable genetic system. Teratog Carcinog Mutagen 1982; 2:19-30.

31. Areces LB, Kazanietz MG, Blumberg PM. Close similarity of baculovirus expressed n-chimaerin and protein kinase C α as phorbol ester receptors. J Biol Chem 1994; 269:19553-19558.

32. Birchall AM, Bishop J, Bradshaw D, Cline A, Coffey J, Elliott LH, Gibson VM, Greenham A, Hallam TJ, Harris W, Hill CH, Hutchings A, Lamont AG, Lawton G, Lewis EJ, Maw A, Nixon JS, Pole D, Wadsworth J, Wilkinson SE. Ro-32-0432, a selective and orally active inhibitor of protein kinase C prevents T-cell activation. J Pharmacol Exp Ther 1994; 268:922-929.

AAS 47
Inflammation:
Mechanisms and Therapeutics
© 1995 Birkhäuser Verlag Basel

REGULATION OF α6β1 INTEGRIN-MEDIATED MIGRATION IN MACROPHAGES

L.M. Shaw and A.M. Mercurio

Laboratory of Cancer Biology
New England Deaconess Hospital and Harvard Medical School
Boston, MA, USA

SUMMARY: Several integrin α subunits have structural variants that are identical in their extracellular and transmembrane domains but that differ in their cytoplasmic domains. In the present study, we examined the possibility that the A and B variants of the α6β1 integrin laminin receptor differ in function. P388D$_1$ macrophages that had been transfected with the α6A integrin subunit were 3-4 fold more migratory than P388D$_1$ macrophages that had been transfected with the α6B integrin subunit. Deletion of the α6 cytoplasmic domain markedly inhibited the ability of the α6β1 receptor to promote migration.

INTRODUCTION

The importance of the extracellular matrix for leukocyte function is well-documented. During an inflammatory reaction, leukocytes must initially interact with the subendothelial basement membrane, which contains laminin and collagen Type IV, and subsequently with the stromal extracellular matrix, which is rich in fibronectin and other collagens (1). In addition to providing a substrate that allows leukocytes to adhere and migrate toward an inflammatory stimulus, the extracellular matrix can also modulate other leukocyte functions that are essential for their participation in an immune response. For example, adhesion to the extracellular matrix proteins laminin and fibronectin can modulate both Fc- and complement-mediated phagocytosis by macrophages (2). In addition, adhesion to the extracellular matrix can influence the response of leukocytes to inflammatory cytokines (3). Taken together, these examples highlight the importance of understanding leukocyte interactions with the extracellular matrix. Such interactions are mediated largely by specific β1 and β2 integrin adhesion receptors.

In previous work, we characterized the adhesion of macrophages to the basement membrane glycoprotein laminin. We demonstrated that these cells require cellular activation to adhere to a laminin substratum and that the receptor on the cell surface that mediates this adhesion is the α6β1 integrin (4). The increased adhesive activity of the α6β1 integrin receptor in response to cellular activation is the result of non-quantitative changes in receptor function. The α6β1 integrin can be expressed as two structural variants, α6A and α6B, that are identical in their extracellular and transmembrane domains but that differ in their cytoplasmic domains (5). Several other integrin subunits also have structural variants and the functional significance of any of these variants is unknown. Using PCR analysis, we determined that macrophages express only the α6A structural variant (6). Transfection of both variant subunits into an α6-deficient macrophage cell line, P388D$_1$, indicated that both α6Aβ1 and α6Bβ1 could upregulate their activity in response to cellular activation (6). Deletional analysis demonstrated that the cytoplasmic domain of the α6 subunit is required for regulating the ligand binding function of the α6β1 receptor (7). A logical question that emerged from these studies is whether the α6Aβ1 and α6Bβ1 variants, as well as the α6-ΔCYTβ1 mutant, exhibit differences in their ability to initiate specific cellular functions subsequent to laminin attachment.

In the present study, we observed that P388D$_1$ cells transfected with either the human α6A, α6B, or α6-ΔCYT integrin cDNAs differed markedly in their ability to migrate toward a laminin gradient. These data indicate that specific sequences within the α6A and α6B cytoplasmic domains differentially modulate the functional activity of the α6β1 integrin and suggest that differential expression of the α6A and α6B variants could have important consequences for leukocyte function.

MATERIALS AND METHODS

cDNA Transfections: The human α6A and α6B cDNAs were cloned by PCR and subcloned into the eukaryotic expression vector pRc/CMV as described previously (6). The α6-ΔCYT mutant cDNA was constructed as described previously (7). The pRc/CMV vectors containing either the α6A, α6B, or α6-ΔCYT cDNAs, as well as the vector alone, were transfected into the P388D$_1$ cell line with Lipofectin (Gibco). Neomycin resistant cells were isolated by selective growth in medium containing G418 (0.4 mg/ml; Gibco). The stable transfectants were pooled and populations of cells that expressed the human α6 subunits on the cell surface were isolated by FACS as described previously (6). A human α6 integrin specific mAb, 2B7, was used for this sorting and for subsequent analysis of the transfectants (6). The sorting was repeated sequentially for each transfectant to enrich for homogeneous populations of cells expressing equivalent levels of the transfected α6 subunits on the cell surface.

Migration Assays.   Cell migration assays were performed using 6.5mm Transwell chambers (8um pore size; CoStar). RPMI-H containing 15 ug/ml laminin (0.6ml) or Puck's Saline A containing 25mM Hepes, 0.5mM $MnCl_2$, 0.1mM $CaCl_2$, 1mM L-Glutamine, and 15 ug/ml laminin were added to the bottom well and the filters were coated for approximately 30 minutes at 37°C. Cells were resuspended in the appropriate buffer at a concentration of 10^6/ml and 10^5 cells were added to the top well of the Transwell chambers. After a 24 hr incubation, the cells that had not migrated were removed from the upper face of the filters using cotton swabs, and the cells that had migrated to the lower surface of the filters were fixed in methanol and then stained with a 0.2% solution of crystal violet in 2% ethanol. Migration was quantitated by counting using brightfield optics with a Nikon Diaphot microscope equipped with a 16-square reticle. The surface area of this grid was determined to be $1mm^2$. Five separate fields were counted for each filter. 2B7 was included in some assays at a concentration of 8 ug/ml to examine inhibition of migration.

RESULTS AND DISCUSSION

   Integrin receptors can initiate a number of cellular events subsequent to ligand binding (8). The importance of α subunit cytoplasmic domains in integrin-mediated cell migration was examined in this study. Populations of cells that expressed equivalent levels of cell surface α6 were obtained by FACS using 2B7, a mAb specific for the human α6 integrin subunit. The levels of α6 expression on the cell surface of the transfectants were monitored by FACS analysis, and only populations that expressed equivalents levels were used for comparative experiments. The α6A and α6B transfectants were examined for their ability to migrate toward a laminin substratum using Transwell chambers. These migration assays were performed in the same medium, RPMI-H, that had been used to examine their adhesion (6,7). The results obtained indicated that the α6A and α6B transfectants differed significantly ($p < 0.01$) in their ability to migrate toward a laminin gradient.   As shown in Fig. 1, the α6A transfectants were 3-4 fold more migratory toward laminin than the α6B transfectants in a 24 hr assay.

   PMA did not increase the number of either the α6A or α6B transfectants that migrated toward laminin (Fig. 1). In fact, a slight decrease in the number of cells that migrated was often observed with PMA. This finding is in contrast to the marked increase in adhesion of these transfectants to laminin in response to PMA stimulation that we previously reported (6).   The migration of both the α6A and α6B transfectants is α6β1 dependent because it was completely inhibited by 2B7 under all of the conditions examined (Fig. 1A).

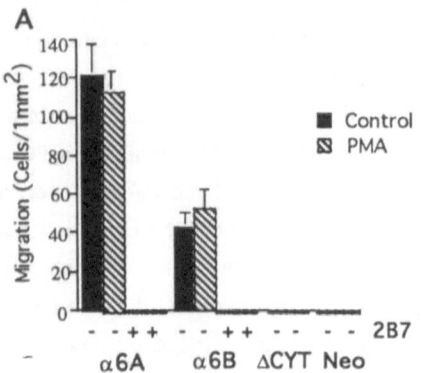
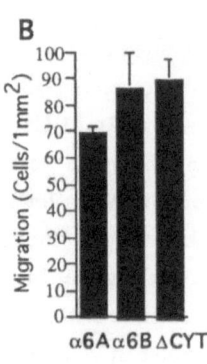

Figure 1. A) Migration of α6A-P388D₁, α6B-P388D₁, and α6ΔCYT-P388D₁ cells toward a laminin substratum. B) Migration of α6A-P388D₁, α6B-P388D₁, and α6ΔCYT-P388D₁ cells toward fetal calf serum.

P388D₁ cells that were transfected with the α6 cytoplasmic deletion mutant, α6-ΔCYT, did not migrate toward laminin under these conditions. This observation is consistent with our previous finding that the α6-ΔCYT transfectants did not adhere to laminin in RPMI-H (7). P388D₁ cells transfected with the pRc/CMV vector alone also did not migrate (Fig. 1A). The difference in migration that was observed for the transfectants was specific for laminin because the α6A, α6B, and α6-ΔCYT transfectants migrated to the same extent when fetal calf serum (15%) was included in the bottom well of the Transwell chamber (Fig. 1B). These results suggest that specific sequences of the α6A and α6B subunit cytoplasmic domains can differentially influence the ability of the α6Aβ1 and α6Bβ1 receptors to promote migration toward a laminin substratum. This finding is important because it is the first report to provide functional significance for the existence of integrin cytoplasmic domain isoforms. The fact that macrophages express only the α6A variant correlates well with their motile phenotype. These mechanistic results substantiate immunohistochemical studies which observed that differential expression of the α6A variant is associated with the induction of migration of both optic neurons (9) and embryonic stem cells (5).

The ability of the α6-ΔCYT transfectants to migrate in normal culture medium cannot be assayed because they do not attach to laminin in the presence of physiological concentrations of Ca^{2+} and Mg^{2+}. Although these mutant transfectants adhere to laminin in the presence of Mn^{2+} (7), the use of this cation is complicated by the fact that Ca^{2+} is required for migration and Ca^{2+} negatively regulates Mn^{2+} adhesion (data not shown). However, conditions were determined that could support the adhesion of the α6-ΔCYT transfectants (0.5 mM Mn^{2+} and 0.1mM Ca^{2+})

at equivalent levels as the wild type α6 transfectants.   Under these conditions, the α6 A transfectants were 2-3 fold more migratory than the α6B transfectants (Fig. 2), a difference similar to that observed in RPMI-H (Fig. 1). Interestingly, the α6-ΔCYT transfectants exhibited some migration toward laminin in the presence of these divalent cations, but the amount of this migration was low in comparison to that observed for the α6A and α6B transfectants (Fig. 2). The differences that were observed for the migration of the α6A and α6B transfectants under both control and PMA conditions are significant ($p < 0.01$). The differences in migration between the α6B and α6-ΔCYT transfectants were not found to be significant ($p > 0.05$).

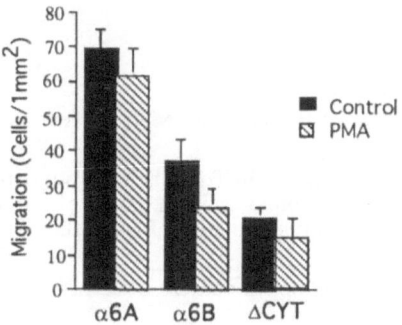

Figure 2. Effect of Mn^{2+} on the migration of the α6A-P388D₁, α6B-P388D₁, and α6ΔCYT-P388D₁ transfectants toward laminin.

The α6 subunit cytoplasmic domain strongly influenced the ability of the α6β1 integrin to mediate migration on laminin. Although the mutant α6ΔCYTβ1 receptor could support adhesion to laminin to the same extent as the wild type receptor in the presence of the divalent cation Mn^{2+}, this mutant receptor was markedly impaired in its ability to mediate migration under the same conditions. Therefore, the α6 cytoplasmic domain must play an important role in α6β1-mediated migration on laminin.

The results obtained in this study raise the question of how integrin subunit cytoplasmic domains influence or signal the post-ligand binding functions of integrin receptors. Motility requires dynamic cytoskeletal associations, and α subunit cytoplasmic domains have been shown to influence the interactions of integrin receptors with cytoskeletal proteins (10). It is possible that α subunit cytoplasmic domains are required to modulate the interactions of β subunit cytoplasmic domains with the cytoskeleton. Therefore, in the absence of the α6 cytoplasmic domain, the β1 cytoplasmic domain may remain more stably associated with the cytoskeleton which would inhibit the dynamic changes that are required for cell migration. In addition, the ability of α subunit cytoplasmic domains to activate unique signal transduction cascades may also contribute to the response of a cell when it binds to laminin (8). Future studies should focus on elucidating the signaling properties of the α6β1 integrin to understand further how the α6 cytoplasmic domain influences cell migration on laminin.

ACKNOWLEDGEMENTS

This work was supported by National Institutes of Health grant CA-42276. L. Shaw was a Ryan Fellow at Harvard Medical School. A. Mercurio is the recipient of an American Cancer Society Faculty Research Award.

REFERENCES

1. Hay, ED., (ed.). Cell Biology of Extracellular Matrix. New York: Plenum Press, 1991.

2. Bohnsack JF, Kleinman HK, Takahashi T, O'Shea JJ, and Brown E. Connective tissue proteins and phagocytic cell function. Laminin enhances complement and Fc-mediated phagocytosis by cultured human macrophages. J Exp Med 1985; 161:912-923.

3. Nathan, C and Sporn M. Cytokines in context. J Cell Biol 1991; 113:981-986.

4. Shaw LM, Messier JM, and Mercurio AM. The activation dependent adhesion of macrophages to laminin involves cytoskeletal anchoring and phosphorylation of the α6β1 integrin. J Cell Biol 1990; 110:2167-2174.

5. Cooper HM, Tamura RN, and Quaranta V. The major laminin receptor of mouse embryonic tem cells is a novel isoform of the α6β1 integrin. J Cell Biol 1991; 115:843-850.

6. Shaw LS, Lotz M, and Mercurio AM. Inside-out integrin signalling in macrophages. Analysis of the role of the α6Aβ1 and α6Bβ1 integrin variants in laminin adhesion by cDNA expression in an α6 integrin deficient macrophage cell line. J Biol Chem 1993; 268:11401-11408.

7. Shaw LM, and Mercurio AM. Regulation of α6β1 integrin laminin receptor function by the cytoplasmic domain of the α6 subunit. J Cell Biol 1993; 123:1017-1025.

8. Hynes RO. Integrins: Versatility, modulation, and signaling in cell adhesion. Cell 1992; 69:11-25.

9. de Curtis I, and Reichardt LF. Function and spatial distribution in developing chick retina of the laminin receptor α6β1 and its isoforms. Development 1993; 118:377-388.

10. Briesewitz R, Kern A, and Marcantonio EE. Ligand-dependent and independent integrin focal contact localization: the role of the α chain cytoplasmic domain. Mol Biol Cell 1993; 4:593-604.

AAS 47
Inflammation:
Mechanisms and Therapeutics
© 1995 Birkhäuser Verlag Basel

NITRIC OXIDE: WHAT ROLE DOES IT
PLAY IN INFLAMMATION AND TISSUE DESTRUCTION?

C.H. Evans

University of Pittsburgh School of Medicine
Ferguson Laboratory - Musculoskeletal Research Center
Pittsburgh, PA USA

SUMMARY: Large amounts of nitric oxide (NO) are produced at sites of inflammation through the action of inducible nitric oxide synthase (iNOS) present in both infiltrating leucocytes and activated, resident tissue cells. However, the role of NO in inflammation remains unclear. NO is a vasodilator, which inhibits the adhesion of neutrophils to the vascular endothelium; it reduces the production of IL-6 by Kupffer cells and chondrocytes, and the production of gamma-IFN and TNF-α by splenocytes. The literature provides contradictory information on the effect of NO on vascular leakiness, chemotaxis, prostaglandin production and tissue damage. Increasingly, data suggest that NO is immunosuppressive. Inhibitors of NOS have potent prophylactic activity in several but not all, animal models of inflammatory disease. However, in rat adjuvant arthritis, therapeutic activity is weak. Whether inhibitors of iNOS will be therapeutically useful in human inflammatory diseases cannot be predicted on the basis of present information.

INTRODUCTION

Nitric oxide (NO) is synthesized by a family of nitric oxide synthases (NOS; EC 1.14.13.39) which oxidatively deiminate the terminal guanidino group of L-arginine to form L-citrulline and NO (reviewed in ref. 1). Molecular oxygen and NADPH are co-substrates. All forms of NOS contain haem, FAD, FMN and tetrahydrobiopterin as prosthetic groups and require calmodulin.

Two so-called "constitutive" isoforms of NOS (cNOS) and one "inducible" form (iNOS) have been purified, cloned and characterized. The two constitutive isoforms are known as "endothelial" NOS (eNOS) and "brain" or "neuronal" NOS (bNOS or nNOS) after the tissues from which they were first isolated. This nomenclature has been challenged partly because recent work is demonstrating a much wider tissue distribution than these names indicate. An alternative nomenclature suggests that bNOS be called NOS-I, iNOS become NOS-II and eNOS, NOS-III.

Important differences exist in the regulation and enzymic activity of cNOS and iNOS. Cells expressing the former isoform rapidly and transiently produce small amounts of NO following exposure to stimuli which raise cytosolic levels of free Ca^{2+}. Cells that can synthesise NO only via the inducible isoform of NOS do not generate NO under basal conditions. Instead, there is a delay of several hours during which the iNOS gene is derepressed. Induction of iNOS usually requires exposure to cytokines, endotoxin or both. Once iNOS has been induced, it produces large amounts of NO for hours or days in a Ca^{2+}-independent manner.

All forms of NOS are inhibited with approximately equal potency by N^G-monomethyl-L-arginine (NMA). N^G-Nitroarginine-methylester (NAME) on the contrary, inhibits cNOS more strongly than iNOS, whereas aminoguanidine has the reverse selectivity.

Constitutive isoforms of NOS are crucial for the maintenance of normal, homeostatic physiology, particularly in the cardiovascular system and brain. Inducible NOS, on the contrary, may be active only under pathophysiological circumstances. This short review addresses one aspect of this, namely the role of NO in inflammation. More extensive discussion of this topic is found in references 2-5.

NO SYNTHESIS IN INFLAMMATION

Both infiltrating leucocytes and activated tissue cells can contribute to the generation of NO at sites of inflammation. Activated rodent neutrophils, lymphocytes, mast cells and, in particular, macrophages (6) produce large amounts of NO. Attempts to induce the synthesis of large amounts of NO by human macrophages *in vitro* have given mixed findings with most authors unable to obtain positive results (reviewed in 7). However, immunohistological staining of human tissues *ex vivo* is beginning to reveal the expression of iNOS in human macrophages *in situ* (8), suggesting that failure to stimulate iNOS expression *in vitro* reflects a failure to arrive at the appropriate culture conditions.

Whether human neutrophils synthesize NO is also controversial (9,10), and there are no data for human lymphocytes or human mast cells. Regardless of the contributions made by leukocytes, it is clear that the resident cells of inflamed tissues are themselves capable of synthesizing large amounts of NO following stimulation by cytokines. Hepatocytes (11), chondrocytes (12) and smooth muscle cells (13), for example, readily express iNOS. This enzyme has been cloned from human hepatocytes and human chondrocytes. As a result of inflammation, levels of NO_3^- are elevated in the blood, urine and local compartments such as synovial fluid.

EFFECTS OF NO ON INDIVIDUAL COMPONENTS OF THE INFLAMMATORY RESPONSE

Inflammation is not a single process, but a complex, multifaceted mosaic of individual events which may differ in their responses to NO. A simplified version of this sequence of events is given in Fig. 1. One of the earliest changes is local vasodilatation which helps account for the heat and redness that are classically associated with inflammation. The endothelial lining becomes leaky, allowing the extravasation of fluid which contributes to oedema. Endothelium also becomes more adhesive, facilitating the binding and subsequent diapedesis of first neutrophils, then monocytes and macrophages and, if an immune reaction is present, lymphocytes. Following extravasation, these cells migrate into the surrounding tissues under the influence of chemotactic stimuli. Leukocytes and resident cells within the inflamed sites then communicate via paracrine and autocrine pathways that result in the production of various mediators which degrade the surrounding tissue and perpetuate and amplify the inflammatory process. Such episodes may resolve, or progress to a chronic inflammatory state.

Table 1. Effects of NO on components of the inflammatory process

Event	Effect of NO
Vasodilatation	↑
Vascular Leak	↑↓
Neutrophil Adhesion	↓
Diapedesis	?
Chemotaxis	↑↓
Mediator Release (also see Table 2)	↑↓

↑ - indicates NO increases; ↓ - indicates NO inhibits; where both appear together, the literature is contradictory; ? -indicates effect unknown

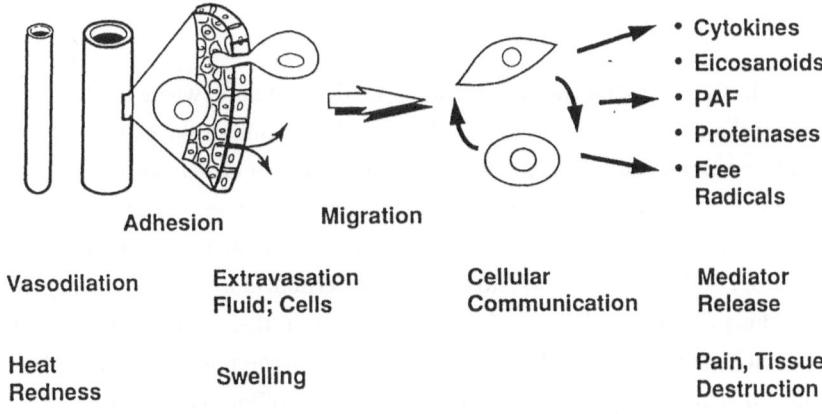

Figure 1. The inflammatory process.

Table 2. Nitric oxide and cytokine release

Cytokine	Cell	Effect of NO
IL-6	Chondrocytes, Kupffer Cells	Inhibition
IL-1	Kupffer Cells	None
TNF-α	Kupffer Cells, Macrophages	None
TNF-α	Splenocytes	Inhibition
Gamma-IFN	Splenocytes	Inhibition

Although there is a reasonably extensive literature describing the effects of NO on the various events depicted in Fig. 1, this literature is confusing and certainly does not permit NO to be categorized simply as a proinflammatory or antiinflammatory molecule. Not only does NO affect different components of the process in different ways, but in several areas the literature is contradictory (Table 1).

Several inhibitory effects of NO on cytokine release (Table 2) should have anti-inflammatory sequelae. Although NO has been reported to activate both constitutive and inducible forms of cyclooxygenase and thus increase prostaglandin production in a number of cell types (14-16), inhibitors of NOS increase PGE_2 synthesis by Kupffer cells (17) and chondrocytes (12). NMA also increases the synthesis of thromboxane B_2 by rat Kupffer cells (17). NO donors inhibit the production of leukotriene B_4, as well as superoxide and β-glucuronidase, by neutrophils (18). The effect of NO on the release of superoxide, PAF and histamine by mast cells is also inhibitory (19,20) and NO has anti-anaphylactic activity (21).

EFFECTS OF NO ON IMMUNE FUNCTION

In rodents, NO has a well established role in non-specific immunity, where the large amounts of NO generated by the iNOS present in activated macrophages inhibit the growth of a variety of microorganisms and tumor cells. Whether this is also the case in humans remains to be seen (7).

The effects of NO on specific immunity, in contrast, have not yet been extensively investigated. The existing data suggest that NO suppresses, rather than enhances, immune function. It inhibits T-cell proliferation, MHC class II expression on mouse peritoneal macrophages (22) and antigen presentation by lung dendritic cells (23). NO has no effect on IL-2 synthesis or the induction of IL-2 receptor. NO has been implicated in tumour-induced immunosuppression (24) and in the reduced immunological response resulting from administration of morphine (25).

The apparent immunosuppressive properties of NO notwithstanding, inhibitors of NOS ameliorate the early events in graft-v-host disease (26), although they fail to increase survival of allografted hearts (278). However, L-NAME lowers T-cell responsiveness in rats with adjuvant arthritis (26). The latter observation conflicts with the data of Gregory et al. (29) showing that NOS inhibitors enhance T-cell responsiveness in mice infected with *Listeria*. However, inhibitors of NOS are potent prophylactic reagents in a variety of immune-driven animal models of disease, several examples of which are to be found in Table 3. It is possible that NO may be essential for certain early events in the immune response, but inhibitory towards later events. Such biphasic behaviour would give NO an important role in regulating the level and duration of the immune response. NO and immune function has been reviewed (30).

NO AND TISSUE DESTRUCTION

Both cells and their extracellular matrices are potentially susceptible to the effects of NO. Cell death, either by necrosis or apoptosis, can occur in response to NO. Paradoxically, there are also suggestions that NO may be protective in, for example, ischaemia-reperfusion.

Whether cells are protected or injured by NO may well hinge on the precise nature of the local chemical reactions that NO undergoes with other free radicals. There is presently much interest in the possible formation of peroxynitrite anion ($ONOO^-$) as a result of a reaction between NO and superoxide. Peroxynitrite, in turn, has the potential to rearrange harmlessly and form nitrate, or to generate the highly reactive hydroxyl and nitrogen dioxide radicals. Although the direct measurement of peroxynitrite is very difficult, it is thought to cause nitrotyrosination of proteins. Nitrotyrosine has been detected immunohistologically in sections of inflamed tissues, and by HPLC in rheumatoid synovial fluids.

Extracellular matrices may be modified directly by NO, or indirectly via effects on their biosynthesis or degradation. Articular cartilage is the best studied tissue in this regard. In response to interleukin-1, articular chondrocytes break down their extracellular matrix at elevated rates while synthesizing new matrix molecules at a reduced rate. NO suppresses the synthesis of cartilage proteoglycans and type II collagen, and is at least partly responsible for the inhibitory effects of IL-1 (31,32). This would suggest a chondroprotective role for NO blockers were it not for the observation that NMA increases proteoglycan release from fragments of bovine cartilage stimulated with IL-1, without affecting the basal level of proteoglycan release (our unpublished data). The mechanisms through which NO modulates matrix metabolism by articular chondrocytes are under investigation. Preliminary data indicate that the addition of NMA to chondrocytes stimulated by IL-1 strongly increases their synthesis of IL-6 and PGE_2 (Hauselmann et al., unpublished).

EFFECTS OF NOS INHIBITORS ON ANIMAL MODELS OF INFLAMMATORY DISEASES

In most cases, inhibitors of NOS show prophylactic activity in animal models of inflammatory diseases (Table 3). Although such studies do not reveal the mechanisms of disease suppression, they do encourage the notion that NO is in some way involved in disease onset. Nevertheless, such an involvement is unlikely to be simple. For instance, although NAME and NMA both inhibit the onset of adjuvant arthritis in rats (28,33), aminoguanidine fails to do so at concentrations which completely suppress the urinary excretion of NO_2^- and NO_3^- (34). Nevertheless, aminoguanidine is active in rat models of diabetes (35).

Another concern is that the impressive prophylactic activity of NMA in adjuvant arthritis is not matched by its therapeutic activity. The ability of NMA to inhibit joint swelling in adjuvant rats falls as the time of administration is delayed and it has only weak activity, at best, in established disease (34).

In one model of hepatitis and in septicaemia, which can be considered as a form of systemic inflammation, NMA exacerbates disease suggesting that NO is protective (36,37). Possible protective mechanisms include the neutralisation of superoxide, anti-thrombotic effects, and the maintenance of organ perfusion by vasodilatation.

Table 3. Effects of NOS inhibitors in inflammation

Species	Disease	Inhibitor	Effect
Rat	Arthritis, (SCW[a])	NMA	Inhibition
Rat	Arthritis	NAME	Inhibition
	(Adjuvant)	NMA	Inhibition
		AG[a]	None
Rat	Diabetes	AG	Inhibition
Mouse	Lupus	NMA	Inhibition
	(MRL/1pr)		
Guinea Pig	Colitis	NAME	Inhibition
Mouse	Encephalomyelitis	AG	Inhibition
Rat	Hepatitis	NMA	Exacerbation
	(LPS + C. Parvum)		
Various	Septicaemia	NMA	Exacerbation

[a]AG = Aminoguanidine; SCW = Streptococcal Cell Wall

POSSIBILITIES OF DRUG DEVELOPMENT

There has been a widespread feeling that highly selective inhibitors of iNOS with the appropriate pharmacokinetic properties would prove to be potent, broad spectrum anti-inflammatory drugs. The information presented in this short review suggests a more cautious approach. Although NO is clearly involved in inflammatory processes, the relationship between NO and inflammation is complex. Not only does NO appear to influence the various components of the inflammatory cascade differently, but its effects may vary with time, concentration and according to the ambient physiological conditions. NO may be anti-inflammatory under certain circumstances and proinflammatory under others. Moreover, acute inflammation may respond differently from chronic inflammation.

Development of novel drugs based upon the manipulation of NO production or activity will require much further, detailed studies of the ways in which NO affects individual inflammatory events in well defined, specific disease entities.

REFERENCES

1.   Knowles RG, Moncada S. Nitric oxide synthases in mammals. Biochem J 1994; 298:249-258.

2.   Nussler AK, Billiar TR. Inflammation, immunoregulation, and inducible nitric oxide synthase. J Leuko Biol 1993; 54:171-178.

3.   Morris SM, Billiar TR. New insights into the regulation of inducible nitric oxide synthesis. Am J Physiol 1994; 266:E829-E839.

4.   Evans CH, Stefanovic-Racic M, Lancaster J. Nitric oxide and its role in orthopaedic disease. Clin Orthop Rel Res in press, 1994.

5.   Evans CH. Nitric oxide and inflammation In: The Immune Consequences of Trauma, Shock and Sepsis. Mechanisms and Therapeutic Approaches. Faist E, editor. Springer-Verlag, 1994: in press

6.   Hibbs JB, Taintor RR, Vavoin Z, Rachlin EM. Nitric oxide, a cytotoxic activated macrophage effector molecule. Biochem Biophys Res Commun 1988; 157:87-94.

7.   Denis M. Human monocytes/macrophages: NO or no NO? J Leuko Biol 1994; 55:682-684.

8.   Kobzik L, Bredt DS, Lowenstein CJ, Drazen J, Gaston B, Sugarbaker D, Stamler JS. Nitric oxide synthase in human and rat lung: immunocytochemical and histochemical localization. Am J Respir Cell Mol Biol 1993; 9:371-377.

9.   Wright CD, Mulsch A, Busse R, Oswald H. Generation of nitric oxide by human neutrophils. Biochem Biophys Res Comm 1989; 160:813-819.

10.   Yan L, Vandivier RW, Suffidini AF, Danner RL. Human polymorphonuclear leukocytes lack detectable nitric oxide synthase activity. J Immunol 1994; 153:1825-1834.

11.   Billiar TR, Curran RD, Stuehr DJ, Stadler J, Simmons RL, Murray SA. Inducible cytosolic enzyme activity for the production of nitrogen oxides from L-arginine in hepatocytes. Biochem Biophys Res Comm 1990; 168:1034-1040.

12.   Stadler J, Stefanovic-Racic M, Billiar TR, Curran RD, McIntyre LA, Georgescu HI, Simmons RL, Evans CH. Articular chondrocytes synthesize nitric oxide in response to cytokines and lipopolysaccharide. J Immunol 1991; 147:3915-3920.

13.   Koide M, Kawahara Y, Tsuda T, Yokoyama M. Cytokine-induced expression of an inducible type of nitric oxide synthase gene in cultured vascular smooth muscle cells. FEBS Lett 1993; 318:213-217.

14.   Salvemini D, Misko TP, Masferrer JL, Seibert K, Currie MG, Needleman P. Nitric oxide activates cyclooxygenase enzymes. Proc Natl Acad Sci USA 1993; 90:7240-7244.

15.   Corbett JA, Kwon G, Turk J, McDaniel ML. IL-1β induces the coexpression of both nitric oxide synthase and cyclooxygenase by islets of langerhans: activation of cyclooxygenase by nitric oxide. Biochemistry 1993; 32:13767-13770.

16.   Inoue T, Fukuo K, Morimoto S, Koh E, Ogihara T. Nitric oxide mediates interleukin-1 induced prostaglandin production by vascular smooth muscle cells. Biochem Biophys Res Commun 1993; 194:420-424.

17.   Stadler J, Harbrecht BG, DiSilvio M, Curran RD, Jordan ML, Simmons RL, Billiar TR. Endogenous nitric oxide inhibits the synthesis of cyclooxygenase products and interleukin-6 by rat Kuppfer cells. J Leuko Biol 1993; 53:165-172.

18.   Moilanen E, Vuorinen P, Kankaanranta H, Metsa-Ketela T, Vapaatalo H. Inhibition by nitric oxide donors of human polymorphonuclear leucocyte functions. Br J Pharmacol 1993; 109:852-58.

19.   Hogaboam CM, Befus AD, Wallace JL. Modulation of rat mast cell reactivity by IL-1_. Divergent effects on nitric oxide and platelet-activating factor release. J Immunol 1993; 151:3767-3774.

20.   Mannaioni PF, Masini E, Pistelli A, Salvemini D, Vane JR. Mast cells as a source of superoxide anions and nitric oxide-like factor relevance to histamine release. Int J Tissue React 1991; 13:271-278.

21.   Masini E, Gambassi F, DiBelli MG, Mugnai L, Raspani S, Mannaioni PF. Nitric oxide modulates cardiac and mast cell anaphylaxis. Agents Actions 1994; 41:C89-C90.

22.   Sicher SC, Vazquez MA, Lu CY. Inhibition of macrophage Ia expression by nitric oxide. J Immunol 1994; 153:1293-1300.

23.   Holt PG, Oliver J, Bilyk N, McMenamin C, McMenamin PG, Kraal G, Thepen R. Downregulation of antigen presenting cell function(s) of pulmonary dendritic cells *in vivo* by resident alveolar macrophages. J Exp Med 1993; 177:397-407.

24.   Lejeune P, Lagadec P, Onier N, Pinard D, Ohshima H, Jeannin JF. Nitric oxide involvement in tumor-induced immunosuppression. J Immunol 1994; 152:5077-5083.

25.   Fecho K, Maslonek KA, Coussons-Read ME, Dykstra LA, Lysle DT. Macrophage-derived nitric oxide is involved in the depressed concanavalin A responsiveness of splenic lymphocytes from rats administered morphine *in vivo*. J Immunol 1994; 752:5845-5852.

26.   Garside P, Hutton AK, Severn A, Liew FY, Mowat AM. Nitric oxide mediates intestinal pathology in graft-vs-host disease. Eur J Immunol 1992; 22:2141-2145.

27.   Bastian NR, Xu S, Shao XL, Shelby J, Granger DL, Hibbs JB. N^G-monomethyl-L-arginine inhibits nitric oxide production in murine cardiac allografts but does not affect graft rejection. Biochim Biophys Acta 1994; 1226:225-231.

28.   Ialenti A, Moncada S, DiRosa M. Modulation of adjuvant arthritis by endogenous nitric oxide. Br J Pharmacol 1993; 110:701-706.

29.   Gregory SH, Wing EJ, Hoffman RA, Simmons RL. Reactive nitrogen intermediates suppress the primary immunologic response to Listeria. J Immunol 1993; 150:2901-2909.

30.   Langrehr JM, Hoffman RA, Lancaster JR, Simmons RL. Nitric oxide - a new endogenous immunoregulator. Transplantation 1993; 55:1205-1212.

31.   Taskiran D, Stefanovic-Racic M, Georgescu HI, Evans CH. Nitric oxide mediates suppression of cartilage proteoglycan synthesis by interleukin-1. Biochem Biophys Res Comm 1994; 200:142-148.

32.   Hauselmann H, Oppliger L, Michel BA, Stefanovic-Racic M, Evans CH. Nitric oxide and proteoglycan biosynthesis by human articular chondrocytes in alginate culture. FEBS Lett 1994; 352:361-364.

33.   Stefanovic-Racic M, Meyers K, Meschter C, Coffey JW, Hoffman RA, Evans CH. N-monomethyl arginine, an inhibitor of nitric oxide synthase, suppresses the development of adjuvant arthritis in rats. Arthritis Rheum 1994; 37:1062-1069.

34.   Stefanovic-Racic M, Meyers K, Meschter C, Coffey JW, Hoffman RA, Evans CH. Comparison of the nitric oxide synthase inhibitors methylarginine and aminoguanidine as therapeutic and prophylactic agents in rat adjuvant arthritis. submitted.

35.   Wang JL, Sweetland MA, Lancaster JR, Williamson JR, McDaniel ML. Aminoguanidine, a novel inhibitory of nitric oxide formation, prevents diabetic vascular dysfunction. Diabetes 1992; 41:552-556.

36.   Billiar T, Curran R, Harbrecht D, Stuehr D, Denetris A, Simmons R. Modulation of nitrogen oxide synthesis *in vivo*: N^G-monomethyl-L-arginine inhibits endotoxin-induced nitrite/nitrate biosynthesis while promoting hepatic damage. J Leuko Biol 1990; 48:565-569.

37. Cobb JP, Natanson C, Hoffman WD, Lodato R, Banks S, Koev C, Solomon M, Elin J, Hosseini J, Danner R. N^W-amino-L-arginine, an inhibitor of nitric oxide synthase raises vascular resistance but increases mortality rates in awake canines challenged with endotoxin. J Exp Med 1992; 176:1175-1189.

AAS 47
Inflammation:
Mechanisms and Therapeutics
© 1995 Birkhäuser Verlag Basel

REGULATION OF FUNCTION AND EXPRESSION OF P-SELECTIN

Rodger P. McEver

W. K. Warren Medical Research Institute and Departments of Medicine and Biochemistry, University of Oklahoma Health Sciences Center, and Cardiovascular Biology Research Program, Oklahoma Medical Research Foundation, 825 N.E. 13th St., Oklahoma City, OK 73104, USA

SUMMARY: P-selectin is an adhesion receptor for leukocytes that is expressed on activated platelets and endothelial cells. The surface expression of P-selectin is tightly regulated through signals in the cytoplasmic domain that mediate sorting into secretory granules, internalization into coated pits, and targeting to lysosomes for degradation. Like the other selectins, P-selectin binds sialylated, fucosylated carbohydrate ligands such as sialyl Lewis x. However, it binds with much higher affinity to PSGL-1, a sialomucin-like glycoprotein on myeloid cells. Binding of PSGL-1 to P-selectin may be essential for leukocytes to roll on P-selectin-expressing cells under shear forces.

INTRODUCTION

The selectins (E-, L-, and P-selectin) are three related adhesion receptors that mediate the initial rolling adhesion of leukocytes to the vessel wall by binding to carbohydrate ligands on apposing cells. Since their cloning in 1989, the selectins have been the subject of intense study because of their predicted important roles in both physiological and pathological inflammation. Earlier work on the selectins has been reviewed ((1) and references therein). This paper discusses recent studies of P-selectin.

RESULTS AND DISCUSSION

P-selectin is constitutively synthesized by megakaryocytes and venular endothelial cells, where it is sorted into secretory granules: the α granules of platelets and the Weibel-Palade bodies of endothelial cells. Upon stimulation by agonists such as thrombin and histamine, P-selectin is rapidly redistributed to the cell surface, where it mediates adhesion of leukocytes. On activated endothelial cells, P-selectin is rapidly internalized. The cytoplasmic domain of P-selectin contains the information required for sorting into secretory granules (2) as well as for internalization into clathrin-coated pits (H. Setiadi and R. P. McEver, unpublished observations). Antibody-tagging studies suggest that a portion of P-selectin can be resorted into new Weibel-Palade bodies after internalization, although the techniques used were not quantitative (3). In transfected cells lacking secretory granules, P-selectin has a very short half-life because a signal in its cytoplasmic domain directs rapid movement from endosomes to lysosomes, where it is degraded (4). Collectively, these data indicate that sorting signals in the cytoplasmic domain serve to limit the expression of P-selectin on the cell surface. Certain cytokines also increase the synthesis of P-selectin in endothelial cells both in vitro and in vivo (5). The 5' flanking region of the human P-selectin gene has been cloned (6), but further studies are required to determine how inflammatory mediators augment transcription of the gene. Cytokine-induced increased synthesis of P-selectin may saturate the sorting pathway to secretory granules, resulting in expression of P-selectin on the cell surface in the absence of degranulation. A second stimulus leading to degranulation might further augment the levels of P-selectin on the cell surface.

Many small sialylated, fucosylated, and (in some cases) sulfated oligosaccharide ligands for the selectins have been described, of which the prototype is the tetrasaccharide, sialyl Lewis x. However, these ligands bind with very low affinity to the selectins. In contrast, a single glycoprotein in myeloid cell extracts binds with relatively high affinity to P-selectin (7). This ligand, a minor component of the plasma membrane glycoproteins, is an extensively sialylated dimer consisting of two disulfide-linked subunits of M_r 120,000. It has many sialylated, clustered O-linked glycans that render it susceptible to cleavage with the enzyme O-sialoglycoprotein endopeptidase (8). Consistent with these properties, the cDNA-derived amino acid sequence of the ligand, now termed P-selectin Glycoprotein-1 (PSGL-1), indicates that it is a type I membrane protein with an extracellular domain rich in serines, threonines, and prolines, characteristics of mucin-like molecules (9). A recombinant form of PSGL-1, co-expressed in COS cells with a fucosyltransferase, mediates adhesion to E- and P-selectin-expressing cells. Many of the O-linked glycans on the recombinant PSGL-1 appear to be simple type I chains that can be removed with sialidase and O-glycanase (9). In contrast, native PSGL-1 from human neutrophils is largely resistant to cleavage with O-glycanase, and has at least some complex O-linked glycans that include poly-N-acetyllactosamine terminating in the sialyl Lewis x structure (10). Native PSGL-1 also binds to E-selectin, but with 50-fold lower affinity than to P-selectin (10). The structures of the oligosaccharides and, perhaps, their sites of attachment to the polypeptide chain will need to be determined to understand why PSGL-1 binds so well to P-selectin. Comparative studies will be required to ascertain the degree to which the glycosylation, and hence the function, of recombinant PSGL-1 resembles that of the native molecule on leukocytes.

Myeloid cells treated with O-sialoglycoprotein endopeptidase no longer adhere to P-selectin, even though the total surface expression of sialyl Lewis x is unchanged (8). This result suggests, but does not conclusively establish, that PSGL-1 play a critical role in adhesion of myeloid cells to P-selectin. We have recently prepared monoclonal antibodies to PSGL-1, one of which blocks binding of purified PSGL-1 to P-selectin. The monoclonal antibodies should prove to be valuable reagents for defining the biological significance of PSGL-1 for adhesion of leukocytes to P-selectin, particularly under the shear forces characteristic of postcapillary venules.

REFERENCES

1. McEver RP. Selectins. Curr Opin Immunol 1994;6:75-84.

2. Disdier M, Morrissey JH, Fugate RD, Bainton DF, McEver RP. Cytoplasmic domain of P-selectin (CD62) contains the signal for sorting into the regulated secretory pathway. Mol Biol Cell 1992; 3:309-321.

3. Subramaniam M, Koedam JA, Wagner DD. Divergent fates of P- and E-selectins after their expression on the plasma membrane. Mol Biol Cell 1993; 4:791-801.

4. Green SA, Setiadi H, McEver RP, Kelly RB. The cytoplasmic domain of P-selectin contains a sorting determinant that mediates rapid degradation in lysosomes. J Cell Biol 1994; 124:435-448.

5. Weller A, Isenmann S, Vestweber D. Cloning of the mouse endothelial selectins. Expression of both E- and P-selectin is inducible by tumor necrosis factor. J Biol Chem 1992; 267:15176-15183.

6. Pan J, McEver RP. Characterization of the promoter for the human P-selectin gene. J Biol Chem 1993; 268:22600-22608.

7. Moore KL, Stults NL, Diaz S, Smith DL, Cummings RD, Varki A, McEver RP. Identification of a specific glycoprotein ligand for P-selectin (CD62) on myeloid cells. J Cell Biol 1992; 118:445-456.

8. Norgard KE, Moore KL, Diaz S, Stults NL, Ushiyama S, McEver RP, Cummings RD, Varki A. Characterization of a specific ligand for P-selectin on myeloid cells. A minor glycoprotein with sialylated O-linked oligosaccharides. J Biol Chem 1993; 268:12764-12774.

9. Sako D, Chang X-J, Barone KM, Vachino G, White HM, Shaw G, Veldman GM, Bean KM, Ahern TJ, Furie B, Cumming DA, Larsen GR. Expression cloning of a functional glycoprotein ligand for P-selectin. Cell 1993; 75:1179-1186.

10. Moore KL, Eaton SF, Lyons DE, Lichenstein HS, Cummings RD, McEver RP. The P-selectin glycoprotein ligand from human neutrophils displays sialylated, fucosylated, O-linked poly-N-acetyllactosamine. J Biol Chem 1994; 269:22318-22327.

AAS 47
Inflammation:
Mechanisms and Therapeutics
© 1995 Birkhäuser Verlag Basel

REGULATION OF L-SELECTIN EXPRESSION BY MEMBRANE PROXIMAL PROTEOLYSIS

Takashi K. Kishimoto, Julius Kahn, Grace Migaki, Elizabeth Mainolfi, Francine Shirley, Richard Ingraham, and Robert Rothlein

Boehringer Ingelheim Pharmaceuticals, Inc., Ridgefield, CT. USA 06877.

SUMMARY: L-selectin is a lectin cell adhesion molecule expressed on the cell surfaces of lymphocytes, monocytes and granulocytes. Upon leukocyte activation or L-selectin cross-linking the transmembrane-bound L-selectin is rapidly shed from the cell surface. Based on these observations, it has been proposed that L-selectin is proteolytically cleaved from the cell surface. However a panel of common protease inhibitors have no effect on L-selectin proteolysis. To further define the mechanism of L-selectin down-regulation we have produced reagents to study proteolytic fragments of L-selectin. We have developed a trapping ELISA for the detection of soluble L-selectin. In addition we have produced a high affinity polyclonal antisera against the extracellular domain and against the cytoplasmic domain of L-selectin. Both antisera immunoprecipitate the intact form of L-selectin from metabolically labeled PHA lymphoblasts and peripheral blood neutrophils. We review here our progress in defining a 6 kD L-selectin transmembrane peptide (L-STMP) from PMA activated lymphoblasts and fMLP-activated neutrophils. Radiochemical sequencing data indicate that the cleavage site occurs between Lys[321] and Ser[322] in a short membrane-proximal region of the extracellular domain.

INTRODUCTION

L-selectin is a member of the selectin adhesion family, which includes E-selectin and P-selectin (reviewed in 1-3). The selectins are involved in guiding leukocyte traffic to sites of inflammation. L-selectin is expressed on the cell surfaces of lymphocytes, monocytes, and granulocytes (4). On lymphocytes, L-selectin serves primarily to mediate tissue specific migration of lymphocytes to peripheral lymph nodes (1,2). Neutrophil adhesion to IL-1-stimulated HUVEC is partially L-selectin-dependent (5,6). In vivo neutrophil migration to inflamed skin or peritoneum can be blocked by anti-L-selectin MAb (4,7) and by an L-selectin-IgG chimera (8). L-selectin has been shown to be involved in neutrophil rolling along endothelial cells both in vitro and in vivo (5,9,10).

L-selectin is rapidly downregulated on neutrophils and lymphocytes exposed to activating agents (7, 11-14). A large fragment of L-selectin, corresponding to most of the extracellular domain, can be recovered from the supernatant of activated neutrophils (11). The shedding event is extremely rapid, occurring concurrently with the rapid upregulation of the Mac-1 integrin (11). It has been proposed that chemotactic agents provide a trigger for the transition from L-selectin-mediated neutrophil rolling and initial binding to the ß$_2$ integrin-mediated firm adhesion and transendothelial migration (7,11). More recently, Jutila and colleagues have found that cross-linking of the surface L-selectin results in its shedding (15). They have proposed that normal leukocyte trafficking and rolling may result in continuous shedding of L-selectin from the cell surface. Western blot analysis provided suggestive evidence for activation-independent shedding in vivo (15).

A proteolytic mechanism could be defined by either identifying inhibitors against a specific class of protease which have activity against L-selectin downregulation or by identifying cleavage products of L-selectin. In this review we summarize our experience with screening panels of protease inhibitors for activity against L-selectin downregulation and in producing reagents to isolate cleavage products. We have raised a polyclonal antiserum against a synthetic peptide corresponding to the cytoplasmic domain of L-selectin. We have previously demonstrated that this antiserum can recognize the intact form of L-selectin as well as a 6 kD transmembrane fragment of L-selectin associated with activated leukocytes and L-selectin transfectants.

MATERIALS AND METHODS

Cell and serum isolation. Human peripheral blood was collected in heparin, and PBMC and granulocytes were isolated using dextran sedimentation followed by Ficoll-Paque (Pharmacia, Uppsala, Sweden) gradient. PBMC were activated with 100 ng/ml PMA for 30 min at 37˚C and granulocytes were activated with 10^{-7} M FMLP for 30 min at 37˚C. For serum collection, normal human blood was collected into sterile vacutainers, and the blood was allowed to clot for at least 0.5 h before collection of serum.

Monoclonal antibodies. Mouse mAbs (Dreg-55, -56, -110, -200 and -152) directed against L-selectin were prepared as previously described (14).

Polyclonal antisera. A polyclonal antiserum against the extracellular domain of L-selectin was generated by hyperimmunization of a rabbit with a purified preparation of a soluble, truncated form of L-selectin, as previously described. A polyclonal antiserum against the cytoplasmic domain of L-selectin was generated by hyperimmunization of a rabbit with a BSA-conjugated 18mer synthetic peptide corresponding to the entire cytoplasmic domain of L-selectin with an additional N-terminal cysteine residue (NH$_2$-CRRLKKGKKSKRSMNDPY-COOH), as previously described (19).

Metabolic labeling.   Human mononuclear leukocytes were isolated from peripheral blood by ficoll-hypaque centrifugation and dextran sedimentation, as described previously (14). PHA-stimulated lymphoblasts were generated by incubating the mononuclear leukocytes with 2.5 µg/ml PHA (Sigma) in complete RPMI-1640 medium for 5 days at 37°C. The PHA lymphoblasts were harvested on day 5 and metabolically labeled with [^{35}S]-methionine as described previously.

Immunoprecipitation and SDS-PAGE. Cell lysates were precleared with normal rabbit serum followed by protein A-agarose. One micoliter of preimmune serum or specific serum was added to aliquots of the precleared lysates and cell-free supernatants. The samples were incubated at 4°C for 1 - 2 h and then 15 ml of a protein A-agarose slurry was added to each sample. Samples were rotated end-over-end at 4°C for 30 min and then washed extensively. The specifically bound material was eluted by addition of SDS-PAGE sample buffer followed by incubation at 90 °C for 10 min. Eluates were resolved on tricine-SDS polyacrylamide gradient (10-20%) gels (NOVEX). Gels were subjected to fluorography (Enhance, NEN) and autoradiography.

Immunofluorescence and flow cytometry. Leukocytes were incubated with 20 µg/ml MAb in phosphate buffered saline containing 2% rabbit serum for 30 min at 4°C, as previously described (14). The cells were washed three times and stained with a phycoerythrin-conjugated F(ab')$_2$ fragments of goat anti-mouse IgG for 30 min at 4°C. The cells were washed and fixed in paraformaldehyde prior to analysis on a Becton Dickinson FACScan.

Recombinant soluble L-selectin. The sequence encoding the signal sequence and extracellular domain of human L-selectin was amplified by PCR from a full-length L-selectin cDNA clone (generous gift of B. Seed (16)). The soluble L-selectin construct was cloned into the CDM8 expression vector (16) and expressed in COS cells by DEAE-Dextran transfection as described previously (16). Supernatant from the transfectants were collected on days 3 - 12 and assayed for L-selectin by ELISA.

cL-selectin ELISA assay. Anti-L-selectin mAb Dreg 55, (2.5 µg/ml) was added to 96 well flat bottom E.I.A. microtiter plates (Linbro) at 50 ul/well at room temperature for 1 hour. Wells were washed three times with DPBS and then blocked with 200 ul of 2% BSA-DPBS for 1 h at 37°C. Wells were flicked empty and a titration of standard sera (two-fold dilutions 1:4-1:32) and serum samples (diluted in 1% BSA-DPBS) were added (50 µl/well) in duplicate for 1 h at 37°C. Wells were washed three times with DPBS. The biotinylated anti-L-selectin mAb (Dreg 200) was added at 0.63 µg/ml (50 µl/well) for 30 minutes at 37°C. Wells were washed three times with DPBS. Horseradish peroxidase conjugated streptavidin (Zymed, San Francisco, CA) (1:4000) was added (50 µl/well) for 30 minutes at 37°C. Wells were washed three times with DPBS and once with ABTS substrate buffer (Zymed). ABTS substrate was then added (50 µl/well) and the plates were read on a Molecular Devices reader (410 nm) until maximum OD readings were obtained. Mean

OD readings were calculated and the sL-selectin concentrations were calculated from the standard sera titration.

RESULTS

L-selectin down-regulation is resistant to protease inhibitors. A panel of common protease inhibitors, representing inhibitors of the four basic categories of proteases, was tested for their ability to inhibit L-selectin downregulation on fMLP-activated neutrophils. As a control for specifity, neutrophils were also analyzed for Mac-1 expression. Mac-1 is stored in intracellular granules which are mobilized upon neutrophil activation and result in a dramatic upregulation of Mac-1 surface expression. Protease inhibitors were tested for their ability to inhibit L-selectin downregulation without affecting Mac-1 upregulation. Table 1 summarizes our results with inhibitors of serine proteases (PMSF, APMSF, aprotinin, antipain, chymostatin, leupeptin,TLCK,TPCK, 3,4-dichloroisocoumarin), metalloproteases (EDTA, phosporamidon, bestatin, leupeptin), aspartic proteases (pepstatin) and cysteine proteases (E64). None of these protease inhibitors at a wide range of concentrations had any specific effect on L-selectin down-

Table 1 The effects of protease inhibitors on L-selectin and Mac-1 expression on fMLP-activated neutrophils

Inhibitor	Class of protease	Concentration	L-selectin	Mac-1
Antipain	serine	10-100 µg/ml	no effect	no effect
APMSF	serine	10 - 80 µg/ml	no effect	no effect
Aprotinin	serine	2 - 20 µg/ml	no effect	no effect
Bestatin	metallo	10 - 80 µg/ml	no effect	no effect
Chymostatin	serine	20 - 200 µg/ml	no effect	no effect
DCI	serine	10 - 50 µg/ml	no effect	no effect
E64	cysteine	100 - 1000 µg/ml	no effect	no effect
EDTA	metallo	2 - 10 mM	no effect	no effect
Leupeptin	serine	0.1 - 1 µg/ml	no effect	no effect
Pepstatin	aspartic	0.15 - 1.5 µg/ml	no effect	no effect
Phosphoramidon	metallo	20 - 330 µg/ml	no effect	no effect
TPCK	serine	3.5 - 35 µg/ml	no effect	inhibits
TLCK	serine	3.5 - 35 µg/ml	no effect	no effect

regulation. Interestingly TPCK inhibited Mac-1 upregulation without affecting L-selectin downregulation, suggesting that these two events involve independent signalling pathways.

ELISA assay for the detection of sL-selectin. We developed a sandwich ELISA for the detection of the soluble form of L-selectin (sL-selectin). The DREG series of MAb was originally generated against the shed form of L-selectin (14), and thus were good candidates to test for use in an ELISA assay. DREG-55, -56, -110, -152, and -200 were absorbed to polystyrene microtiter wells. Neutrophils were activated at 10^7/ml with 10^{-6} M fMLP to induce shedding of the L-selectin. Supernatant from activated PMN was added to the MAb-coated wells. The trapped L-selectin was detected with biotinylated DREG-200 MAb. The combination of the DREG-55 capture MAb and the DREG-200 detecting MAb gave the highest specific signal. Substitution of anti-ICAM-1 RR1/1 MAb as either the trapping MAb or the biotinylated detecting MAb resulted in complete loss of activity (data not shown). In order to quantify the levels of soluble L-selectin, a

A

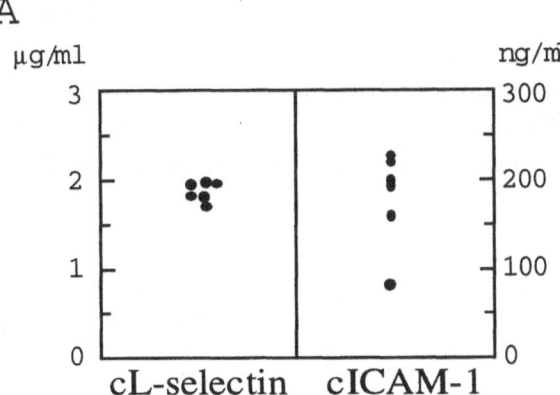

Figure 1.   A) cL-selectin and cICAM-1 levels in normal sera. Serum from six healthy adults was collected, serially diluted, and levels of cL-selectin and cICAM-1 were quantitated by ELISA. B) Levels of cICAM-1 but not cL-selectin increase significantly in a variety of inflammatory disease states. Serum from patients with systemic lupus erythromatosis, Kawasaki's disease, sepsis, rheumatoid arthritis and burn was collected and analyzed by ELISA for cL-selectin and cICAM-1 levels.

B

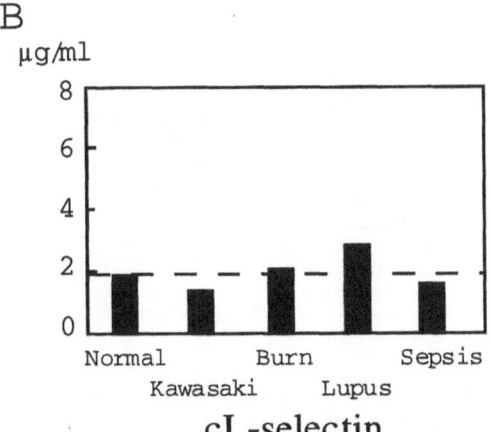

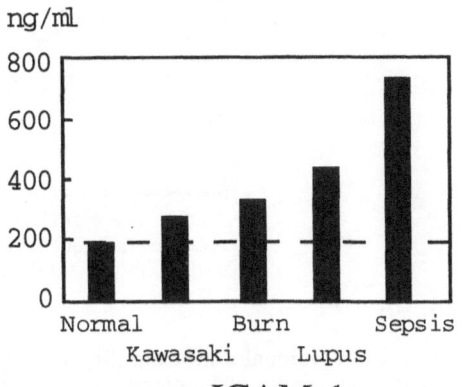

recombinant sL-selectin cDNA construct, lacking the transmembrane and cytoplasmic domains, was produced. Detection of serial dilutions of the purified molecule indicated a lower limit of 170 ng/ml sensitivity. Normal human serum has a high basal level of a circulating form of soluble L-selectin (1.9 +/- 0.11 µg/ml) compared to a range of 0.176 +/- 0.054 µg/ml of cICAM-1 in the same individuals (Figure 1A), which is in good agreement with previously published values (17,18). The level of ICAM-1 has been shown to be elevated in a variety of disease states. We compared levels of cL-selectin versus cICAM-1 in normal sera and in sera from patients with Kawasaki's disease, SLE, burn, and sepsis (Figure 1B). A baseline of cICAM-1 and cL-selectin in normal individuals was established. In all disease states examined there was a significant increase in the levels of cICAM-1. In patients with sepsis the levels of cICAM-1 was increased 4-fold (736 +/- 375 ng/ml). In marked contrast, the levels of cL-selectin remained relatively constant in all diseases studied.

<u>Identification of L-selectin cleavage products.</u> We raised two antisera against L-selectin, one directed against purified soluble L-selectin lacking the transmembrane and cytoplasmic domains (sera JK923), and another directed against a synthetic peptide corresponding to the entire cytoplasmic domain of L-selectin (JK564), as described previously (19) (Fig. 2). JK923specifically stains intact, unactivated leukocytes, while JK564 stains only permeabolized cells (data not shown). Both antisera immunoprecipitated the intact membrane-spanning form of

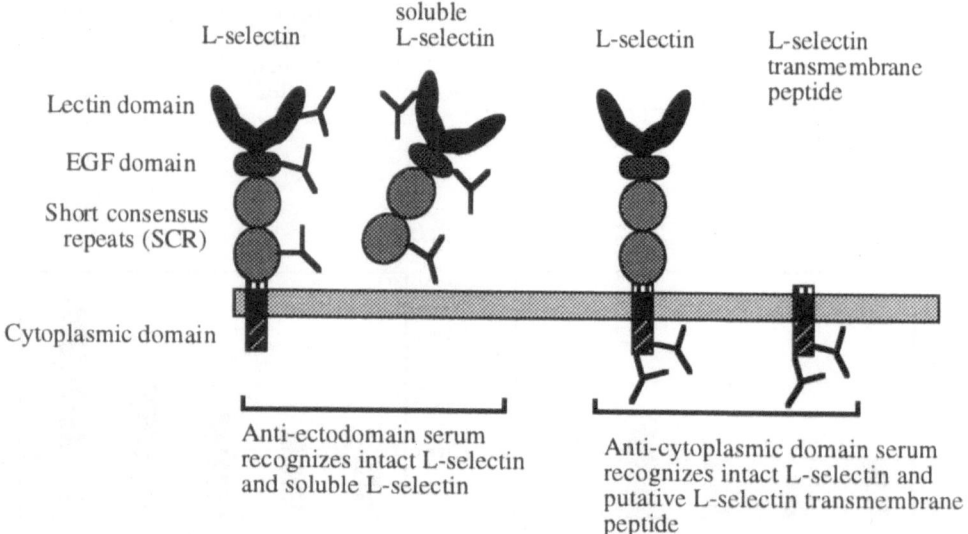

Figure 2. Polyclonal antiserum directed against the extracellular domain of L-selectin and the cytoplasmic domain of L-selectin. Both antiserum react with native transmembrane L-selectin. The anti-ectodomain serum also reacts with soluble L-selectin, while the anti-cytoplasmic domain serum reacts with the L-selectin transmembrane peptide fragment.

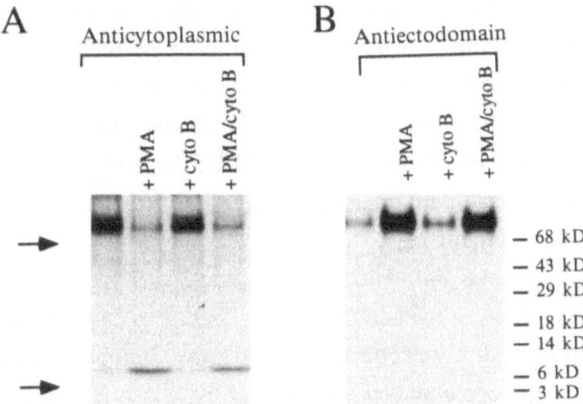

Figure 3.   Identification of L-selectin cleavage products from metabolically labeled PHA lymphoblasts.   Peripheral blood lymphocytes were stimulated with PHA for   five days. Lymphoblasts were pulse-labeled with [^{35}S] -methionine for 15 min, chased with cold methionine for 30 min, and then treated with PMA (100 ng/nl) for 30 min, as indicated.   A) Labeled cells were lysed in 1% Triton X-100 solution, and cell lysates were immunoprecipitated with antiserum directed against the cytoplasmic domain of L-selectin. The upper arrow denotes the position of the native form of L-selectin; the lower arrow denotes the position of the 6 kD transmembrane cleavage product. B) Cell-free supernatants were immunoprecipitated with antisera against the ectodomain serum. The arrow denotes the position of the soluble form of L-selectin. Immunoprecipitates were subjected to SDS-PAGE on 10-20% gradient gels and visualized by autoradiography with fluorography. (Reprinted from Kahn et al, 1994, J. Cell Biol. (19))

L-selectin (Fig. 3 and data not shown). We next asked whether we could detect processed fragments of L-selectin on activated leukocytes with these antisera. The primary sequence of L-selectin predicts six methionine residues, two of which are located in the cytoplasmic and transmembrane domains. A third methonine residue is located in the ectodomain, 10 amino acids proximal to the beginning of the transmembrane domain. We reasoned that both a transmembrane fragment of L-selectin as well as a soluble form of L-selectin should be detectable in cells metabolically labeled with [^{35}S]-methionine. At day 5, PHA-stimulated lymphoblasts actively synthesize L-selectin. The anti-ectodomain serum immunoprecipitated the intact 70 kD L-selectin molecule from biosynthetically labeled cells (Fig. 3). Although PHA blasts are activatively proliferating and constitutively which induced a significant increase in the downregulation of cell surface L-selectin. This is evidenced by reduced levels of intact L-selectin in immunoprecipitates from cell lysates (Fig 3A), increased levels of soluble L-selectin in immunopreciptates from cell-free supernatants (Fig 3B), and decreased cell surface expression of L-selectin (data not shown). The anti-cytoplasmic domain serum also recognizes the intact form of L-selectin (Fig. 3A), but not the soluble form (data not shown). These results indicate that the classical transmembrane form of

L-selectin is the major species found on these cells, and that the soluble form of L-selectin lacks the cytoplasmic tail. In addition, a faint band of 6 kD can be reproducibly detected with the anti-cytoplasmic domain serum in cell lysates of day 5 PHA blasts. Activation with phorbol esters caused a marked decrease in the amount of detectable 70 kD intact L-selectin and a corresponding marked increase in the amount of the 6 kD species. These data suggest that the 70 kD intact L-selectin species is processed upon activation with phorbol esters to yield a 6 kD cell bound fragment and a 65 kD soluble fragment.

Identification of the cleavage site. The actual cleavage site was determined by N-terminal radiochemical sequence analysis of the 6 kD L-STMP product, as described previously (19). The lysates of PHA lymphoblasts or L-selectin-transfected COS cells biosynthetically labeled with [^{35}S]-methionine were immunoprecipitated with the anti-cytoplasmic domain serum, subjected to SDS-PAGE, and transferred to PVDF membrane. The 6 kD band was visualized by autoradiography, excised and subjected to protein sequencing. Radioactive peaks were observed at cycles 4 and 20, indicating methionine residues at these positions. A spacing of 16 amino acids between the two methionine residues is found only between Met^{325} and Met^{341} of the L-selectin sequence, suggesting that L-selectin was cleaved between Lys^{321} and Ser^{322}. To confirm thispredicted cleavage site, we performed radiochemical sequence analysis with cells biosynthetically labeled with another radiolabeled amino acid, [^{3}H]-phenylalanine. Radioactive peaks were observed at cycles 2, 14, and 24, indicating phenylalanine residues at these sites. The spacing between the observed peaks was consistent only with the spacing between Phe^{323}, Phe^{335}, and Phe^{345} of L-selectin, again indicating a cleavage site between Lys^{321} and Ser^{322} (Figure 3).Cleavage at this site would produce a transmembrane peptide with a predicted molecular mass of 5823 daltons, which is in excellent agreement with the observed Mr = 6 kD by SDS-PAGE.

DISCUSSION

The two step adhesion model, which depicts neutrophil rolling mediated by selectins, followed by neutrophil exposure to chemokines, and finally neutrophil transendothelial migration mediated by the β_2 integrins is widely accepted (20). However within the context of this model it remains unclear why or if L-selectin needs to be downregulated. We originally postulated that L-selectin downregulation may be necessary for neutrophils to progress from initial contact to transendothelial migration (11). Alternatively L-selectin downregulation may serve as a protective mechanism to prevent neutrophils activated in circulation from entering an inappropriate tissue site. More recently, Jutila et al. (15) showed that crosslinking of L-selectin causes downregulation of L-selectin, and proposed that shedding of L-selectin may be a continuous process during neutrophil

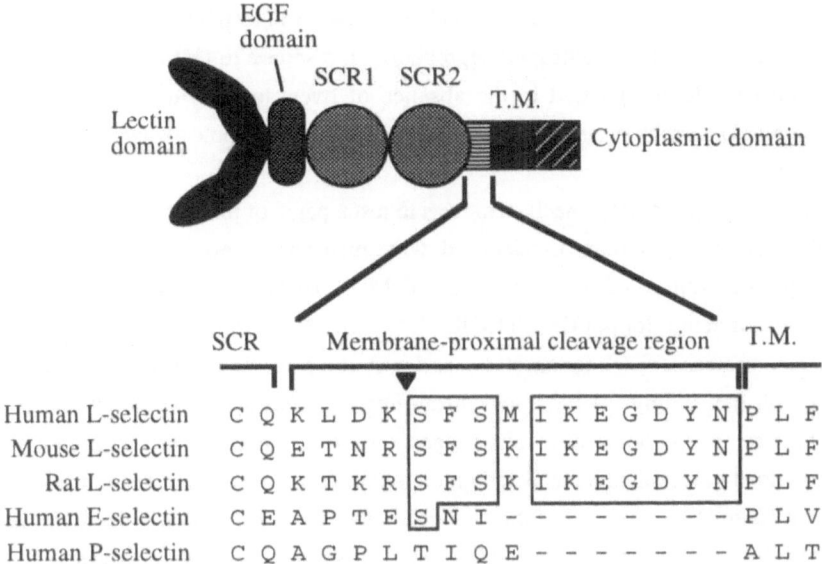

Figure 4. The 6 kD species is an L-selectin transmembrane peptide (L-STMP). Sequence of the membrane-proximal cleavage region of human L-selectin aligned with the corresponding regions of mouse and rat L-selectin and human E-selectin and P-selectin. Conserved residues in this region are boxed, and the C-terminus of the last SCR domain and the N-terminus of the transmembrane domain are indicated. The triangle marks the putative cleavage site between Lysine[321] (K) and Serine[322] (S). (Reprinted from Kahn et al., 1994, J. Cell Biol. (19))

rolling and normal leukocyte trafficking. The continuous shedding of L-selectin during leukocyte trafficking and neutrophil rolling in response to subclinical stimuli may account in part for the high levels of circulating L-selectin in normal serum (18). The finding that cultured neutrophils actively synthesize L-selectin suggests the possibility that at least some of the neutrophil L-selectin can be replenished by de novo synthesis. Although the biological significance of L-selectin downregulation remains to be resolved, it is clear that this is an unusual and precisely regulated processing event.

Downregulation of L-selectin on leukocytes is triggered by specific cell activating agents. These studies indicate that either a protease is mobilized or activated or that L-selectin undergoes a conformational change and becomes accessible to a constitutively active protease. Newly synthesized L-selectin on PHA lymphoblasts and cultured neutrophils still require an activating agent, such as PMA, for efficient L-selectin downregulation, even though these cells are already stimulated to some degree. Daily and colleagues (21) reported that L-selectin downmodulation in response to PMA activation is inhibited by staurosporine, an inhibitor of protein kinase C. However this is not entirely unexpected since PMA directly activates PKC. It is possible that L-selectin downregulation may also occur via PKC-independent pathways in response to chemotactic factors, as has been shown in the case of neutrophil aggregation in response to fMLP versus PMA (22). L-selectin can also be downregulated in the absence of overt leukocyte activation by crosslinking of L-selectin (15), as may occur when L-selectin is crosslinked upon engagement with its endothelial cell ligand.

Our first attempt to define a proteolytic mechanism was to test a panel of protease inhibitors for activity against L-selectin downregulation. L-selectin downregulation appears to be remarkably insensitive to a battery of inhibitors of serine proteases (PMSF, APMSF, aprotinin, antipain, bestatin, dichloroisocoumarin, leupeptin, TLCK, TPCK), metalloproteases (EDTA, phosporamidon), cysteine proteases (E64, iodoacetate), and aspartic proteases (pepstatin) . These results are consistent with the findings of Bazil and Strominger (23), who tested a similar large panel of protease inihbitors. These negative results suggest either a novel protease or a protease that is activated or mobilized so rapidly upon cell activation that these inhibtors have no significant effect on L-selectin downregulation. Recently Jutila and colleagues provided evidence that DFP, a potent serine protease inhibitor, can inhibit L-selectin release from activated leukocytes and L-selectin-crosslinked leukocytes.   Other leukocyte membrane proteins, including CD14 (24), CD16 (25), CD43 (26-28), CD44 (28), and TNF receptor (29,30), have been reported to be downmodulated upon leukocyte activation. However the rapid kinetics of L-selectin shedding is unusual. A soluble form of ICAM-1 (17) has been reported in the supernatant of stimulated lymphocytes and monocytes over a period of hours to days, although the precise mechanism to generate this soluble form is unknown. CD43 and CD44 on neutrophils are downregulated over a period of 15 min - 60 min in response to PMA (27), but this is in contrast to the cleavage of L-selectin within minutes on the same cells. Moreover physiological stimuli, such as TNF and fMLP are poor modulators of CD43 and CD44 cleavage, but cause efficient downregulation of L-selectin (26). CD16 (FcgRIII) is expressed as both a PI-linked form (CD16-I) on neutrophils and a transmembrane bound form (CD16-II) on NK cells. Both forms are released upon cell activation; however, release of CD16-II, but not CD16-I, appears to involve a proteolytic mechanism (25). CD14 is also a PI-linked protein, although release of CD14 appears to involve a proteolytic mechanism (24). A cDNA encoding a PI-linked form of L-selectin has been reported (6); however, L-selectin expression is not deficient in patients lacking PI-linked proteins (31). Common serine protease inhibitors, such as PMSF and aprotinin, have been shown to inhibit release of CD14 and CD44 (24,28), while a metalloprotease inhibitor, 1,10 phenanthroline, inhibits release of CD16-II (25). Interestingly, downregulation of CD43 appears to be sensitive to both serine and metalloprotease inhibitors (26-28). These findings indicate that mechanisms that regulate L-selectin proteolysis may be distinct from that of most other leukocyte surface antigens.

To further define a proteolytic mechanism, we sought to identify proteolytic fragments of L-selectin. It has been known that a large fragment of L-selectin can be recovered from the supernatant of activated leukocytes (11,21). We have developed an ELISA to detect cleaved L-selectin, similar to that described by Schleiffenbaum et al (18). Our estimate of the levels of circulating L-selectin (1.9 µg/ml) in normal sera is in good agreement with published reports (18) (1.6 µg/ml). The high levels of cL-selectin in normal sera suggest that L-selectin may be continuously released from leukocytes of healthy individuals. Recent work of Jutila and colleagues demonstrates that crosslinking of L-selectin on the cell surface of unactivated leukocytes results in shedding of L-selectin (15). They further propose that normal trafficking of leukocytes results in crosslinking of L-selectin via its endothelial cell ligand, which in turn causes continuous shedding of L-selectin (15 and M. Jutila, personal communication). Western blot analysis of human plasma provided supportive evidence for L-selectin shedding in vivo (15). It has been estimated that the adult body contains on the order of 10^{12} lymphocytes, with 10^9 new lymphocytes entering the circulation each day. A large portion of these lymphocytes are continuously circulating between lymphoid organs via the blood and lymph. Lymphocytes enter the lymph nodes via specialized high endothelial venules. L-selectin mediates traffic of lymphocytes to peripheral lymph nodes through recognition of a ligand expressed by the HEV. It has been estimated that lymphocytes spend an average of two days in any given lymphoid organ, thus lymphocytes are constantly migrating (1,2). Similarly neutrophil rolling along endothelial surfaces is an L-selectin-dependent event (5,9,10). This rolling behavior along with transient adhesive events may also result in shedding of small amounts of L-selectin. The turnover of neutrophils in normal individuals is enormous: it is estimated that approximately 10^{11} neutrophils are produced each day, with an average lifespan of 2-3 days. If the model proposed by Jutila et al. is correct, the high volume of normal leukocyte traffic and turnover could easily account for the generation of high levels of cL-selectin. The lack of a detectable increase in cL-selectin levels during inflammation may reflect the basal level of cL-selectin that is so high that even a severe inflammatory state, such as sepsis, has little impact on the total amount of cL-selectin. Even in an extreme case where all the neutrophils in the blood are systemically activated, the resulting release of L-selectin is calculated to result in only a minute increase in serum cL-selectin levels.

The physiological role of cL-selectin remains to be elucidated. Watson et al. (8) demonstrated that a bivalent L-selectin-IgG chimera can block neutrophil accumulation to sites of inflammation in vivo. They report that as little as 10 µg injected into mice, resulting in a blood level of about 3 µg/ml, gave significant inhibition. However the bivalent form of the L-selectin-IgG chimera is likely to have a 10-fold higher avidity than the monomer (similar to the difference measured in the avidity of a whole antibody vs an Fab fragment). More recently, Schleiffenbaum et al. (18) reported that the partially purified soluble form of L-selectin can partially inhibit lymphocyte binding to endothlium in vitro at 1.5 µg/ml with maximal inhibition at 12 -15 µg/ml. They speculate that the cL-selectin may serve as a biological adhesion buffer system to prevent excessive leukocyte-endothelial cell interaction. However it is also possible that the local concentration of cL-selectin at an inflammatory site could be quite high and play a significant role in attentuating leukocyte traffic. Alternatively it is possible that the cL-selectin has a role unrelated to adhesion, much like complement fragments have diverse physiological functions. These aspects of cL-selectin warrant further investigation. The high basal level of cL-selectin in normal sera has other clinical significance. Recently there has been an intense effort to identify and develop antagonists of L-selectin for clinical use. However the application of any L-selectin-binding antagonist must take into account the large reservoir of cL-selectin which might tie up a large portion of the antagonist before therapeutic concentrations are achieved.

We have also identified a 6kD L-selectin transmembrane peptide (L-STMP) fragment of L-selectin with a polyclonal antiserum directed against the cytoplasmic tail of L-selectin. A second polyclonal serum directed against the membrane-proximal extracellular region of L-selectin also reacts with the L-STMP product, confirming this is a bonafide transmembrane peptide. N-terminal radiochemical sequence analysis of the 6 kD L-STMP further defines the cleavage site between Lys^{321} and Ser^{322}. This small region between the last short consensus repeat (SCR) and the transmembrane domain is highly conserved between species. However this region is not well conserved with the corresponding regions of E- and P-selectin molecules, which is consistent with the fact that E- and P-selectin are not regulated in the same manner as L-selectin. The lysine at the P1 position is suggestive of a trypsin-like activity; however, L-selectin proteolysis is insensitive to TLCK and other trypsin inhibitors. Further mutagenesis studies will be required to define the specificity of L-selectin proteolysis.

ACKNOWLEDGEMENTS

Sera from Kawasaki patients and from systemic lupus erythromatosus patients were the kind gift of Dr. K. Barron (Texas Children's Hospital, Houston, TX). Sera from burn patients were from Drs.C. Baxter and W. Mileski (University of Texas Southwestern Medical Center, Dallas, TX). Sera from Sepsis patients were the generous gift of Dr. M. Mariscalco (Baylor College of Medicine Houston, TX).

REFERENCES

1. Butcher EC. The regulation of lymphocyte traffic. Curr Topics Microbiol Immunol 1986; 128:85-122.

2. Yednock TA,Rosen SD. Lymphocyte Homing. Adv Immunol 1989; 44:313-378.

3. Lasky LA. Selectins: Interpreters of cell-specific carbohydrate information during inflammation. Science 1992; 258:964-969.

4. Lewinsohn DM, Bargatze RF,Butcher EC. Leukocyte-endothelial cell recognition: Evidence of a common molecular mechanism shared by neutrophils, lymphocytes, and other leukocytes. J Immunol 1987; 138:4313-4321.

5. Smith CW, Kishimoto TK, Abbassi O, et al. Chemotactic factors regulate lectin adhesion molecule-1 (LECAM-1)-dependent neutrophil adhesion to cytokine-stimulated endothelial cells in vitro. J Clin Invest 1991; 87:609-618.

6. Spertini O, Luscinskas FW, Kansas GS, et al. Leukocyte adhesion molecule-1 (LAM-1, L-selectin) interacts with an inducible endothelial cell ligand to support leukocyte adhesion. J Immunol 1991; 147:2565-2573.

7. Jutila MA, Rott L, Berg EL,Butcher EC. Function and regulation of the neutrophil MEL-14 antigen in vivo: Comparison with LFA-1 and Mac-1. J Immunol 1989; 143:3318-3324.

8. Watson SR, Fennie C,Lasky LA. Neutrophil influx into an inflammatory site inhibited by a soluble homing receptor-IgG chimaera. Nature 1991; 349:164-167.

9. Von Andrian UH, Chambers JD, McEvoy LM, Bargatze RF, Arfors K-E,Butcher EC. Two-step model of leukocyte-endothelial cell interaction in inflammation: Distinct roles for LECAM-1 and the leukocyte ß integrins in vivo. Proc Natl Acad Sci USA 1991; 88:7538-7542.

10. Ley K, Gaehtgens P, Fennie C, Singer MS, Lasky LA,Rosen SD. Lectin-like cell adhesion molecule 1 mediates leukocyte rolling in mesenteric venules in vivo. Blood 1991; 77:2553-2555.

11. Kishimoto TK, Jutila MA, Berg EL,Butcher EC. Neutrophil Mac-1 and MEL-14 adhesion proteins inversely regulated by chemotactic factors. Science 1989; 245:1238-1241.

12.Griffin JD, Spertini O, Ernst TJ, et al. Granulocyte-macrophage colony-stimulating factor and other cytokines regulate surface expression of the leukocyte adhesion molecule-1 on human neutrophils, monocytes, and their precursors. J Immunol 1990; 145:576-584.

13. Jung TM, Gallatin WM, Weissman IL,Dailey MO. Down-regulation of homing receptors after T cell activation. J Immunol 1988; 141:4110-4117.

14. Kishimoto TK, Jutila MA,Butcher EC. Identification of a human peripheral lymph node homing receptor: A rapidly down-regulated adhesion molecule. Proc Natl Acad Sci USA 1990; 87:2244-2248.

15. Palecanda A, Walcheck B, Bishop DK,Jutila MA. Rapid activation-independent shedding of leukocyte L-selectin induced by cross-linking of the surface antigen. Eur J Immunol 1992; 22:1279-1286.

16. Camerini D, James SP, Stamenkovic I,Seed B. Leu-8/TQ1 is the human equivalent of the Mel-14 lymph node homing receptor. Nature 1989; 342:78-80.

17. Rothlein R, Mainolfi EA, Czajkowski M,Marlin SD. A form of circulating ICAM-1 in human serum. J Immunol 1991; 147:3788-3793.

18. Schleiffenbaum B, Spertini O,Tedder TF. Soluble L-selectin is present in human plasma at high levels and retains functional activity. J Cell Biol 1992; 119:229-238.

19. Kahn J, Ingraham RH, Shirley F, Migaki GI,Kishimoto TK. Membrane proximal cleavage of L-selectin: Identification of the cleavage site and a 6-kD transmembrane peptide fragment of L-selectin. J Cell Biol 1994; 125:461-470.

20. Butcher EC. Leukocyte-endothelial cell recognition: Three (or more) steps to specificity and diversity. Cell 1991; 67:1033-1036.

21. Jung TM,Dailey MO. Rapid modulation of homing receptors (gp90Mel-14) induced by activators of protein kinase C. J Immunol 1990; 144:3130-3136.

22. Merrill JT, Slade SG, Weissmann G, Winchester R,Buyon JP. Two pathways of CD11b/CD18-mediated neutrophil aggregation with different involvement of protein kinase C-dependent phosphorylation. J Immunol 1990; 145:2608-2615.

23. Bazil V,Strominger JL. Metalloprotease and serine protease are involved in cleavage of CD43, CD44, and CD16 from stimulated granulocytes. Induction of cleavage of L-selectin via CD16. J Immunol 1994; 152:1314-1322.

24. Bazil V,Strominger JL. Shedding as a mechanism of down-modulation of CD14 on stimulated human monocytes. J Immunol 1991; 147:1567-1574.

25. Harrison D, Phillips JH,Lanier LL. Involvement of a metalloprotease in spontaneous and phorbol ester-induced release of natural killer cell-associated FcRIII (CD16-II). J Immunol 1991; 147:3459-3465.

26. Bazil V,Strominger JL. CD43, the major sialoglycoprotein of human leukocytes, is proteolytically cleaved from the surface of stimulated lymphocytes and granulocytes. Proc Natl Acad Sci U S A 1993; 90:3792-3796.

27. Rieu P, Porteu F, Bessou G, Lesavre P,Halbwachs-Mecarelli L. Human neutrophils release their major membrane sialoprotein, leukosialin (CD43), during cell activation. Eur J Immunol 1992; 22:3021-3026.

28. Campanero MR, Pulido R, Alonso JL, et al. Down-regulation by tumor necrosis factor-alpha of neutrophil cell surface expression of the sialophorin CD43 and the hyaluronate receptor CD44 through a proteolytic mechanism. Eur J Immunol 1991; 21:3045-3048.

29. Porteu F,Nathan C. Shedding of tumor necrosis factor receptors by activated human neutrophils. J Exp Med 1990; 172:599-607.

30. Kohno T, Brewer MT, Baker SL, et al. A second tumor necrosis factor recptor gene product can shed a naturally occuring tumor necrosis factor inhibitor. Proc Natl Acad Sci U S A 1990; 87:8331-8335.

31. Ord DC, Ernst TJ, Zhou LJ, et al. Structure of the gene encoding the human leukocyte adhesion molecule-1 (TQ1, Leu-8) of lymphocytes and neutrophils. J Biol Chem 1990; 265:

AAS 47
Inflammation:
Mechanisms and Therapeutics
© 1995 Birkhäuser Verlag Basel

TRANSCRIPTIONAL REGULATION OF ENDOTHELIAL CELL ADHESION MOLECULES: A DOMINANT ROLE FOR NF-κB.

C.C. Chen and A.M. Manning

Cell Biology and Inflammation Research, Upjohn Laboratories, Henrietta Street, Kalamazoo, MI 49002, USA

SUMMARY: A growing body of evidence demonstrates that elevated expression of the endothelial cell adhesion molecules E-selectin, VCAM-1 and ICAM-1 at sites of inflammation *in vivo* is due in whole or part to the upregulation of transcription of their respective genes. Pharmacologic antagonism of transcription from these genes may therefore represent a novel approach to the development of anti-inflammatory therapeutics. This paper reviews our current understanding of nuclear factors which act to regulate the transcriptional activity of the E-selectin, VCAM-1 and ICAM-1 genes, and discusses that evidence which suggests that the nuclear transcription factor NF-κB acts as a dominant regulator of transcription from these genes.

The endothelial cell adhesion molecules E-selectin, VCAM-1 and ICAM-1 play an important role in leukocyte adhesion and transendothelial migration at sites of inflammation. In tissues from a wide range of inflammatory disorders, endothelial expression of these molecules has been documented to be elevated in both a temporal and spatial association with inflammatory cell infiltrates (reviewed in 1). An increasing number of reports have demonstrated that the elevated expression of these adhesion receptors is due in whole or part to the upregulation of expression of the genes encoding them (e.g. 2,3). Primary cultured endothelial cells and purified immune mediators, such as monokines, lymphokines and bacterial endotoxin, have been used as a model system in which to investigate the specific mechanisms responsible for the activation of transcription of these genes (1). These studies have identified the presence of binding sites in the promotor regions of the E-selectin, VCAM-1 and ICAM-1 genes which are recognized by discrete nuclear transcription factors. The role of these factors in regulating transcription from these promotors has also been analyzed both by molecular biologic and more recently by pharmacologic approaches.

Transcriptional regulation of the E-selectin gene has been the subject of intense investigations in recent years (4-9). Sequence analysis has revealed the presence of three closely-spaced binding sites for the nuclear transcription factor NF-κB clustered within a 40 bp segment of DNA within the E-selectin promotor (4,5). On the basis of *in vitro* DNA-binding studies, two additional regulatory elements, termed NF-ELAM1 and NF-ELAM2, have also been identified (6). The sequence of the NF-ELAM1 site is identical to the critical portion of the δA element, reported to be a T-cell-specific enhancer, and which can be recognized by members of the cAMP-independent ATF/CREB family of transcription factors (7). The nature of the factor(s) which bind the NF-ELAM2 element has not yet been identified. However, based on the fact that E-selectin promoter-CAT constructs carrying both NF-ELAM2 and NF-κB elements showed reduced transcriptional activity in the absence of cytokine treatment, it has been proposed that the NF-ELAM2 element may be involved in the repression of the basal activity of the NF-κB enhancer in quiescent cells.

That NF-κB plays a dominant role in transcription of the E-selectin gene is unequivocal. Overexpression of the RelA (p65) subunit of NF-κB results in activation of E-selectin promotor activity in the absence of any cytokine stimuli (10). As a corollary, overexpression of the cytoplasmic inhibitor of NF-κB, IκB-α, effectively abolished cytokine-induced E-selectin promotor activity in primary cultured endothelial cells. Results of deletion analyses and systematic site-directed mutagenesis of the E-selectin promoter region demonstrated that deletion or mutation of any one of the three NF-κB sites abolished cytokine-induced transcriptional activity, indicating that all three NF-κB sites are essential for maximal promoter activity following cytokine treatment. Additionally, it has been reported that the three NF-κB sites are sufficient for the maximal response of E-selectin promoter-reporter constructs to TNFα induction (8). This observation differs from previous studies which demonstrated that additional elements further upstream of the NF-κB sites were also required for maximum response to cytokine stimulation (5,7). Specifically, mutation of either the NF-ELAM1 or NF-ELAM2 site resulted in a marked (~85%) reduction of the response to IL-1 induction, suggesting that both sites are needed to achieve maximal transcriptional activity. In addition, mutation of the NF-ELAM1 binding site significantly reduced the ability of overexpressed NF-κB to activate E-selectin promoter activity, indicating that factors binding to the NF-ELAM1 sites may act in concert with NF-κB to enhance cytokine-induced transcription from the E-selectin promoter. Using affinity chromatography and immunoprecipitation techniques, it has been shown that protein-protein interaction occurs between certain ATF factors and the p50 and RelA subunits of NF-κB (6,7). Hence, it is possible that ATF factors may interact with NF-κB to enhance E-selectin transcription by providing an activation surface which can attract RNA polymerase and accessory transcription factors (11). A recent study demonstrated a further level of complexity in NF-κB-mediated activation of the E-selectin gene (9). High-mobility-group protein I(Y) (HMG-IY) was found to bind to three distinct sites in the E-selectin promoter which overlap with the NF-κB sites. Using electrophoretic mobility shift assays, it was demonstrated that the binding affinity of the p50 subunit to the NF-κB sites within the E-selectin promoter is greatly increased by the presence of HMG-I(Y), suggesting that cooperative interactions between these two families of transcription factors may occur during E-selectin promoter activation.

Analysis of the 5'-regulatory region of the human VCAM-1 gene has identified the presence of two juxtapositioned NF-κB recognition sites close to the transcriptional initiation site (12,13). In addition to these recognition sequences, several GATA boxes, as well as sequences resembling the binding sites for AP-1, Oct-1, Oct-2, and members of the *ets* family of proto-oncogenes have been identified. Promotor-reporter studies utilizing deletion mutants have identified the presence of a putative silencer element in this region, and this element has been hypothesized to play a role in repression of VCAM-1 transcription in unstimulated cells (12). Using fusion plasmids containing varying lengths of 5' flanking sequence of the VCAM-1 gene and the CAT reporter gene, it has been shown that the NF-κB and the GATA binding sites are functional elements in the cytokine-induced activation of VCAM-1 transcription. Both NF-κB sites are absolutely required for transcription of the VCAM-1 gene, as alteration or deletion of either one of them completely abolished TNFα-inducible transcription of the VCAM-1 promoter-CAT construct. Results of electrophoretic mobility shift assays indicated that the two NF-κB sites interact with distinct nuclear proteins (13). That NF-κB plays a dominant role in VCAM-1 transcriptional activation is supported by the demonstration that overexpression of RelA alone activates VCAM-1 promotor activity in the absence of cytokine stimulation, and that overexpression of IκB blocks TNFα-induced VCAM-1 transcriptional activity (14). In addition, double-stranded oligonucleotides encoding the NF-κB DNA-binding sequences and referred to as transcription factor decoys (TFDs), when introduced into the cytoplasm of endothelial cells in culture, were capable of preventing NF-κB translocation to the nucleus and VCAM-1 transcriptional activation in response to TNFα (14). Interestingly, a promoter-CAT construct containing the two NF-κB sites was completely inactive when transfected into the Jurkat T lymphocyte-derived cell line, and did not respond to TNFα treatment (12), even though this cell line is known to contain NF-κB and is commonly used for the analysis of other TNFα-responsive promotors, including that for E-selectin. Selective binding of different members of the NF-κB/rel family of transcription factors appears to provide a means for selective activation of gene transcription (15), and therefore it has been proposed that such a mechanism might be responsible for the cell-specific activity of the VCAM-1 promotor.

In contrast to the NF-κB sites, changes in the sequence or removal of the GATA elements within the VCAM-1 promotor only partially decreased TNFα-induced transcriptional activation (12). Maximal responsiveness to cytokine stimulation was observed only when both elements were present. Since the GATA family of transcription factors is known to cooperate with other *trans*-acting factors to regulate transcription, it has been proposed that factors binding to the GATA and the NF-κB sites may interact to generate full VCAM-1 cytokine responsiveness.

The promoter region of the human ICAM-1 gene has been cloned and sequenced by several laboratories (16-18). Computer analyses of these sequences revealed a number of motifs implicated in the regulation and expression of eukaryotic genes, such as TATA boxes, as well as several potential binding sites for nuclear transcription factors, including Sp-1, AP-1, AP-2, AP-3 and NF-κB. In addition, the presence of a putative silencer, which may be involved in tissue specific repression of ICAM-1 gene expression, has been proposed.

Whether any of these transcription factors are involved in the regulation of ICAM-1 transcription is unknown, because direct evidence for binding of these nuclear factors to the 5'-regulatory regions is currently unavailable. However, using a series of deletion mutants derived from an ICAM-1 promoter-luciferase construct, Voraberger *et al.* (18) demonstrated that deletion of the NF-κB site partially reduced TNFα-induced luciferase activity, suggesting that cis-acting element(s) in addition to NF-κB are required for activation of transcription mediated by cytokines.

The studies summarized above have revealed that many different nuclear transcription factors can be demonstrated to bind to the promotors of the E-selectin, VCAM-1 and ICAM-1 genes in endothelial cells. Further studies will be necessary to fully understand how these factors interact to regulate the activity of these promotors in a cytokine-responsive and tissue-specific manner. These studies have, however, defined the nuclear transcription factor NF-κB as a common component of the transcriptional complexes of all these genes. Antagonism of NF-κB DNA binding to these promotors, whether through deletion or mutation of the NF-κB recognition sequences, through overexpression of IκB-α or through introduction of cytoplasmic TFDs, have been reported to prevent the cytokine-induced activation of transcription of one or all of these genes. This data is consistent with the proposal that NF-κB plays a dominant role in the transcriptional activation of these genes. No other nuclear transcription factor thus far identified has been found to possess similar characteristics. NF-κB appears to be unique in that it has been demonstrated to play a primary role in the transcriptional activation of many genes whose expression is associated with a wide range of inflammatory pathologies. In addition to E-selectin, VCAM-1 and ICAM-1, the transcriptional activation of genes encoding pro-inflammatory cytokines and growth factors including TNFα, IL-8, IL-6, IL-2 and monocyte chemoattractant protein-1 (MCP-1), components of the coagulation system, and immunoreceptors associated with T cell-mediated immune functions have all been demonstrated to be regulated in part through the binding of NF-κB (19). The critical role NF-κB appears to play in regulating the expression of endothelial genes playing a central role in leukocyte accumulation and activation at sites of inflammation has led to the suggestion that NF-κB might be considered a "master regulator" of the inflammatory response (20). Further studies are required to validate this paradigm, however, including the demonstration that NF-κB is activated in association with elevated E-selectin, VCAM-1 and ICAM-1 gene expression at sites of inflammation *in vivo*. Such a demonstration will be the prelude to pharmacologic studies aimed at determining whether inhibition of NF-κB activity can modulate the expression of these proteins and suppress inflammation in animal models of human disease. The paradigm of NF-κB as a master regulator of inflammation predicts that pharmacologic antagonists of NF-κB activation or function would display broad anti-inflammatory activities. Development of small-molecule antagonists of NF-κB function will require a better understanding of the mechanisms regulating the activity of NF-κB in endothelial cells, a subject we and others have recently reviewed (19, 20).

REFERENCES

1. Carlos T, Harlan JM. Leukocyte-endothelial interactions. Blood 1994, 84: 1765-1792.

2. Kukielka GL, Hawkins HK, Michael LH, Manning AM, Lane CL, Entman ML, Smith CW, Anderson DC. Regulation of intercellular adhesion molecule 1 (ICAM-1) in ischemic and reperfused myocardium. J Clin Invest 1993; 92: 1504-1512.

3. Fries JW, Williams AJ, Atkins RC, Newman W, Lipscomb MF, Collins T. Expression of VCAM-1 and E-selectin in an in vivo model of endothelial activation. Am J Path 1993; 143: 725-737.

4. Collins T, Williams A, Johnston GI, Kim J, Eddy R, Shows T, Gimbrone MA, Bevilacqua MP. Structure and chromosomal location for the gene for endothelial-leukocyte adhesion molecule 1. J Biol Chem 1991; 266: 2466-2473.

5. Whelan J, Ghersa P, van Huijsduijnen RH, Gray J, Chandra G, Talbot F, DeLamarter JF. An NF-κB-like factor is essential but not sufficient for cytokine induction of endothelial elukocyte adhesion molecule 1 (ELAM-1) gene transcription. Nucleic Acids Res 1991; 19: 2645-2653.

6. van Huijsduijnen RH, Whelan J, Pescini R, Becker-Andre M, Schenk A-M, DeLamarter JF. A T-cell enhancer cooperates with NF-κB to yield cytokine induction of E-selectin gene transcription in endothelial cells. J Biol Chem 1992; 267: 22385-22391.

7. Kaszubska W, van Huijsduijnen RH, Ghersa P, DeRaemy-Schenk A-M, Chen BP, Hai T, DeLamarter JF, Whelan J. Cyclic AMP-independent ATF family members interact with NF-κB and function in the activation of the E-selectin promoter in response to cytokines. Molec Cell Biol 1993; 13: 7180-7190.

8. Schindler U, Baichwal VR. Three NF-κB binding sites in the human E-selectin gene required for maximal tumor necrosis factor alpha-induced expression. Molec Cell Biol 1994; 14: 5820-5831.

9. Lewis H, Kaszubska W, DeLamarter JF, Whelan J. Cooperativity between two NF-κB complexes, mediated by high-mobility-group protein I(Y), is essential for cytokine-induced expression of the E-selectin promoter. Molec Cell Biol 1994; 14: 5701-5709.

10. Read MA, Whitley MZ, Williams AJ, Collins T. NF-κB and IκBα: an inducible regulatory system in endothelial activation. J Exp Med 1994; 179: 503-512.

11. Tjian R, Maniatis T. Transcriptional activation: a complex puzzle with few easy pieces. Cell 1994; 77: 5-8.

12. Iademarco MF, McQuillan JJ, Rosen GD, Dean DC. Characterization of the promoter for vascular cell adhesion molecule-1. J Biol Chem 1992; 267: 16323-16329.

13. Neish AS, Williams AJ, Palmer HJ, Whitley MZ, Collins T. Functional analysis of the human vascular cell adhesion molecule 1 promoter. J Exp Med 1992; 176: 1583-1593.

14. Shi HB, Agranoff A, Nabel EG, Leung K, Neish AS, Collins T, Nabel G. Differential regulation of vascular cell adhesion molecule-1 gene expression by specific NF-κB subunits in endothelial and epithelial cells. Mol Cell Biol 1994; 13: 6283-6290.

15. Perkins ND, Schmid RM, Duckett CS, Leung K, Rice NR, Nabel G. Distinct combinations of nuclear factor-kappa B subunits determine the specificity of transcriptional activation. Proc Natl Acad Sci USA 1992; 89: 1529-1534.

16. Degitz K, Li LJ, Caughman SW. Cloning and characterization of the 5'-transcriptional regulatory region of the human intercellular adhesion molecule 1 gene. J Biol Chem 1991; 266: 14024-14030.

17. Voraberger G, Schafer R, Stratowa C. Cloning of the human gene for intercellular adhesion molecule 1 and analysis of its 5'-regulatory region. J Immunol 1991; 147: 2777-2786.

18. Cornelius LA, Taylor JT, Degitz K, Li LJ, Lawley TJ, Caughman SW. A 5' portion of the ICAM-1 gene confers tissue-specific differential expression levels and cytokine responsiveness. J Invest Dermatol 1993; 100: 753-758.

19. Baeurle PA, Henkel T. Function and activation of NF-κB in the immune system. Ann Rev Immunol 1994; 12: 141-179.

20. Manning AM, Anderson DC. Transcription factor NF-κB: an emerging regulator of inflammation. In: Annual Reports in Medicinal Chemistry. Bristol JA, editor. San Diego: Academic Press, 1994: 235-244.

AAS 47
Inflammation:
Mechanisms and Therapeutics
© 1995 Birkhäuser Verlag Basel

GENE TARGETING FOR INFLAMMATORY CELL ADHESION MOLECULES

D.C. Bullard, E. T. Sandberg, K. Scharffetter-Kochanek and A. L. Beaudet

Department of Molecular and Human Genetics, Baylor College of Medicine, and Howard
Hughes Medical Institute, Houston, Texas 77030

SUMMARY: Using gene targeting in mouse embryonic stem cells, it is possible to introduce diverse mutations into specific genes. Using these methods, various laboratories have reported mutations for a variety of inflammatory cell adhesion molecules including CD18, α5 integrin, ICAM-1, P-selectin, and L-selectin; preliminary reports of other mutations are also available. Mutations in CD18 and ICAM-1 cause impaired inflammatory and immune responses, mutations in P-selectin and L-selectin cause decreased leukocyte rolling and emigration, and a mutation in α5 integrin causes embryonic lethality. Gene targeting complements other approaches for analyzing the function of inflammatory cell adhesion molecules.

INFLAMMATORY CELL ADHESION MOLECULES

The emigration of leukocytes from the vascular space into the tissues is an important aspect of any inflammatory response. Neutrophils, B lymphocytes, T lymphocytes, monocytes, and other leukocytes display distinct properties, and inflammatory responses differ according to the involved tissue and the nature of the stimulus. These adhesive interactions are mediated by numerous inflammatory cell adhesion molecules (CAM) whose general properties have been reviewed (1-5). These CAMs are members of protein families and include the integrins, immunoglobulin (Ig) family members, selectins, mucin-like proteins, and others. All of the CAM discussed here are type 1 transmembrane proteins with extracellular adhesion domains, transmembrane domains, and cytoplasmic tails. The β2 integrins are heterodimers of a common β (CD18) subunit and differing α (CD11) subunits. The Ig family members include ICAM-1, ICAM-2, VCAM-1, and PECAM-1. The three known selectins (P-, E-, and L-selectin) all contain a Ca^{2+}-dependent lectin binding domain, an EGF-like domain, and a series of complement regulatory domains in addition to the transmembrane domain and cytoplasmic tail. Mucin-like proteins include CD34, GlyCAM-1, and P-selectin glycoprotein ligand (PSGL-1), while MAdCAM-1 reveals homology to both Ig and mucin-like proteins.

The process of leukocyte emigration in postcapillary venules involves multiple steps including leukocyte rolling, firm adhesion, activation, and transmigration with many complexities within each phase of the process. There is strong evidence that leukocyte rolling is mediated largely by the selectins with expression of L-selectin on leukocytes and P- and E-selectin on endothelial cells. The selectins bind to carbohydrate moieties on selectin ligand molecules including CD34 and GlyCAM-1 for L-selectin and PSGL-1 for P-selectin. With firm adhesion and activation, L-selectin is shed from the surface of leukocytes, and the interaction between integrins on leukocytes and Ig family members on endothelial cells assumes greater importance. PECAM-1 is particularly implicated in transmigration. The expression and function of inflammatory CAMs are highly regulated with major effects mediated by inflammatory cytokines; see reviews for details (1-5). Regulatory mechanisms include rapid mobilization of presynthesized protein to the cell surface, increased rates of protein synthesis, changes in cycling of molecules from the cell surface to other cellular compartments, rapid shedding from the surface in the case of L-selectin, and activation to a more adhesive conformation in the case of leukocyte integrins.

The inflammatory CAMs presumably play important roles in cell traffic in the normal healthy state. Neutrophils enter and exit the circulation on a regular basis in the absence of disease. Surveillance against infection at mucosal surfaces presumably relies on regular contributions from these processes. Lymphocytes normally traffic in a very complex pattern through spleen, mesenteric lymph nodes, peripheral lymph nodes, and the vasculature, and there is evidence that this lymphocyte traffic depends on distinct patterns of CAM expression. These CAMs also exert influence on immunological responses through control of lymphocyte traffic and by affecting leukocyte-leukocyte interactions, (e.g., interaction between antigen presenting cells and lymphocytes). It is likely that variation in the expression of these CAMs, whether naturally occurring or pharmacologically induced, could impact on the susceptibility and progression of many human diseases which have a major inflammatory component.

GENE TARGETING

Much of the current knowledge regarding inflammatory CAMs stems from the development of monoclonal antibodies which frequently provided the first definition of the existence for individual CAMs. These antibodies have been used to delineate the pattern of surface expression and to detect responses to inflammatory stimuli; the antibodies were valuable for purification of proteins and cloning of the genes for each CAM. Development of monoclonal antibodies which block adhesive function has contributed the majority of current knowledge regarding the function of individual CAMs, although many other methods such as the use of soluble chimeric proteins have also proven useful. Delineation of the biochemical and molecular basis of leukocyte adhesion deficiency in humans caused by mutations in CD18 (6) provided important insights and reagents as concepts of inflammatory CAMs were evolving. More recently, it is possible to prepare mutations in mice using gene targeting strategies, and mutations in virtually all of the known inflammatory CAMs either have been produced or are being produced.

The strategies for gene targeting were developed in the 1980s and reviews are available (7-10). Embryonic stem (ES) cells can be derived from the inner cell mass of early mouse embryos and maintained in tissue culture. Using techniques for homologous recombination, it is possible to interrupt, delete, or otherwise mutate any cloned mouse gene. The usual first step is to introduce a mutation which totally eliminates the function of a gene (a complete loss of function or "knockout" mutation), although it is possible to introduce virtually any more subtle mutation as discussed below. Once the desired mutation is introduced into the ES cells, these mutated cells are injected into mouse blastocysts resulting in the production of chimeric animals. The chimeric animals can be bred to transmit the mutation to the mouse germline. Transmission from chimeras results in heterozygous mutant mice which may show phenotypic abnormalities, but most mice carrying loss of function mutations in the heterozygous state appear normal despite having half normal levels of the mutated gene product. Heterozygous mice are then bred to produce homozygous animals. Homozygous animals may die in utero, die near the time of birth, show an obvious phenotype, display a subtle phenotype, or appear virtually normal with difficulty detecting any phenotypic variation. The full range of this spectrum has been seen for mice carrying mutations in the various inflammatory CAMs. The gene targeting methodology provides a powerful genetic approach to investigate the function of any gene product and promises to greatly expand the opportunities for studying the role of inflammatory CAMs in normal biology and in diseases processes.

INTEGRINS

A mutation was introduced into the mouse CD18 gene by inserting DNA to create a duplication of exons 2 and 3. Although the intent was to produce a null (complete loss of function) mutation, cryptic promoter activity in plasmid sequences resulted in the production of a hypomorphic (partial loss of function) mutation with the production of low levels of normal protein (11). Homozygous mutant mice are viable and fertile and demonstrate a mild granulocytosis analogous to that seen in human CD18 deficiency. Mutant animals express 2 or 16 percent of normal CD18 levels on the surface of granulocytes in the resting or activated state, respectively. The mutant animals demonstrate an impaired inflammatory response to chemical peritonitis, delayed rejection of cardiac transplants, and impaired delayed type hypersensitivity (11,12). When the CD18 mutation was backcrossed onto a particular (PLJ) inbred mouse background, animals develop a severe inflammatory skin disease which responds dramatically to corticosteroids and is being further investigated (D. C. B. and K. S-K., manuscript in preparation). Our experience with the CD18 mutation demonstrated the importance of carefully designing the DNA construct to introduce a mutation with the desired functional effect. In retrospect, it may prove that the viability of the hypomorphic mutation is quite valuable, and a null mutation is being prepared for comparative analysis. The experience with backcrossing the mutation onto the PLJ strain emphasizes the importance of the basic principle in mouse genetics that many other modifier genes may influence the biology of the primary mutation being studied, and that careful matching of the inbred background of the mouse strain is important in any comparative analysis.

There is a report that a null mutation in the gene for $\alpha 4$ integrin causes embryonic lethality with two distinct defects: failure of allantois to fuse with chorion during placental development and absence of epicardium with lethal cardiac hemorrhage (J. T. Yang, H. Rayburn, R. O. Hynes, submitted manuscript). Mutations in $\alpha 5$ integrin also cause embryonic lethality in homozygotes with mesodermal defects in the embryos (13). The $\alpha 5\beta 1$ integrin functions as a fibronectin receptor, but this integrin is also implicated in cell migration, wound healing, and T cell activation. Mutations in other integrin genes are in preparation in various laboratories.

IMMUNOGLOBULIN FAMILY MEMBERS

There are two reports of mice with mutations in ICAM-1. In one case, a neomycin resistance cassette was used to disrupt exon 5 which encodes Ig domain 4 (14), while the other mutation involved a similar disruption of exon 4 which encodes Ig domain 3 (15). Mice homozygous for either mutation demonstrated normal survival and fertility, profound reduction in expression of ICAM-1, mild granulocytosis, decreased leukocyte emigration with peritonitis, and impaired delayed type hypersensitivity. Mutant cells did not function normally for antigen presentation in the mixed lymphocyte reaction (14), and resistance to the lethal effects of endotoxin or *Staphylococcus aureus* enterotoxin B was demonstrated for mice carrying the exon 4 mutation (15). Subsequent investigations of mice homozygous for the exon 5 mutation (16) have demonstrated residual expression of ICAM-1 related to skipping of the mutated exon. These investigations identified alternative splicing in wild type mice raising the question of whether there may be biologically important alternatively spliced forms of ICAM-1 in wild type mice (16). The skipping of the exon 5 mutation again demonstrates the importance of the precise nature of the mutation relative to the functional effect.

There are preliminary reports of mice with homozygous mutations in VCAM-1 indicating that these animals usually die prenatally, but occasional animals survive (17). It may be possible to prepare mutations in VCAM-1 specific for endothelial cells using methods discussed below, and it can be anticipated that mutant mice will be prepared for other members of the Ig superfamily.

SELECTINS

A null mutation was prepared for P-selectin, and homozygous deficient mice were viable and fertile (18). These mice displayed absence of expression of P-selectin on immunohistochemical analysis, moderate granulocytosis, reduced neutrophil emigration in thioglycolate-induced peritonitis particularly at early time points, and virtual absence of leukocyte rolling in mesenteric venules. Our laboratory also has prepared P-selectin deficient mice displaying a similar phenotype by introducing a mutation which deletes exons 3 to 5 (D.C.B., C. Doerschuk, A.L.B., submitted manuscript). We have bred a line of mice with mutations in both P-selectin and ICAM-1, and observed complete loss of neutrophil emigration into the peritoneum during *Streptococcus pneumoniae*-induced peritonitis at 4 hours, while either mutation alone showed only a 60-70 percent reduction in neutrophil emigration.

Mice carrying a homozygous null mutation in L-selectin were also healthy and viable and showed complete loss of cell surface expression of this CAM (19). These mice showed significant impairment of lymphocyte homing and leukocyte rolling with reduced numbers of lymphocytes in peripheral lymph nodes and reduced neutrophil emigration in thioglycolate-induced peritonitis. A detailed comparison of leukocyte rolling with the published L-selectin deficient mice and the P-selectin deficient mice produced in our laboratory was performed using intravital microscopy to analyze venules of the cremaster muscle in the mouse (20). These studies demonstrated complete absence of rolling in P-selectin mutant mice but normal rolling in L-selectin mutant mice at the earliest time points. At later time points and in TNF-α treated animals, rolling was largely L-selectin dependent.

There are preliminary reports of E-selectin deficient mice indicating that these animals are viable, but no information is available regarding phenotypic abnormalities (17). Our laboratory has recently obtained germline transmission of presumed null mutations for E-selectin and for combined deficiency of E-selectin and P-selectin, but homozygous mutant mice are not yet available (D.C.B., unpublished). Preparation of a double mutation in E-selectin and P-selectin required independent introduction of each mutation onto a single chromosome in ES cells, since double mutants could not be obtained by breeding because these two genes are part of the same cluster and would not show independent assortment. Additional reports of mice with single or multiple mutations in selectins can be anticipated.

OTHER INFLAMMATORY CAMs

Just as monoclonal antibody reagents have been prepared for each of the inflammatory CAMs, it can be anticipated that mutant mice will be produced for each of these molecules and for new molecules yet to be described. Obvious candidates include the CD11 genes, GlyCAM-1, CD34, MAdCAM-1, PECAM-1, and P-selectin glycoprotein ligand as well as additional members of the CAM families discussed above.

THE GENETIC APPROACH

Much of the current knowledge regarding function of inflammatory CAMs stems from studies using monoclonal antibodies or soluble CAMs (frequently Ig-fusion chimeras) to block adhesion. These reagents are particularly useful for *in vitro* studies and are applicable for short term studies *in vivo*. The substantial data already amassed and the ready availability of such reagents provide strong testimony to the power of these methods. However, the availability of mutant mice provides a strong complimentary approach. Mice with homozygous null mutations may be the most definitive test for the contribution of a particular gene product to a biological or disease process. The mutant mice are ideally suited for study of longer term processes or chronic disease models. The effects of half normal levels of gene expression and the combined effects of deficiencies for more than one gene product can be examined relatively readily. The genetic approach and the blocking approach using monoclonal antibodies or soluble proteins both have significant strengths and weaknesses. In most cases, it is likely that data from the two methods of analysis will corroborate the importance of an inflammatory CAM in a particular biological process or disease state. In cases where the data appear to conflict, it will be important to assess the possibility that blocking antibodies or soluble proteins are having effects in addition to abrogating cell adhesion by mechanisms such as interaction with Fc receptors or by inducing cellular responses through cytoplasmic signaling. Any apparent conflicts should also consider the possibility that the mouse mutation may not have created a completely null state or may otherwise differ from the expected functional effect. The importance of the background genotype cannot be overemphasized in mouse experiments. Whether comparing results in a genetic experiment or comparing results between a genetic experiment and a blocking antibody experiment, it is extremely important to consider the possibility that any differences in results might be explained by the use of different inbred strains of mice or the use of mice of mixed background genotype. An obvious disadvantage of the gene targeting methodology at present is the limitation of this technique to mice in comparison to monoclonal antibodies which are generally available for use in other species. Although there could be concern that interpretation of data from mice with congenital mutations might be confused by compensatory responses on the part of other molecules, and it is important to search for such instances, the genetic experience from *E. coli* to man would suggest that such compensatory induction of other systems will be rare. Congenital absence of an inflammatory CAM certainly could influence the development of the immune system and cause a phenotypic effect different from that produced by acute introduction of a blocking monoclonal antibody. These two general strategies should provide complementary information leading to more definitive interpretation of all data, and these methods may also be supplemented by other strategies such as the use of antisense reagents which potentially can be used to induce a deficiency of expression at a later time in the life of an animal.

The gene targeting approach is still being improved in many ways. In addition to the simple knockout mutations, it is possible to introduce virtually any more subtle mutation including single amino acid substitutions, particularly using the "hit and run" or "in and out" strategies (21,22). It is also possible to introduce large duplications of entire genes permitting the analysis of increased dosage which might be important in polygenic disease processes (23). Methods using site specific recombination and recombinase proteins from lower organisms offer the promise of more flexible strategies for gene targeting as exemplified by the *lox*/Cre recombinase system (24). In this system, a functional gene carrying a premutation is introduced, and expression of the Cre recombinase, controlled by a promoter of choice, mediates a recombination event to mutate the gene to a nonfunctional form. These methods offer the potential to introduce mutations in a tissue specific manner using tissue specific promoters to introduce the genetic defect in particular cell types (e.g., perhaps lymphocytes, endothelial cells, or neutrophils in the case of inflammatory CAMs). This strategy might allow, for example, the analysis of the role of VCAM-1 in endothelial cells by circumventing the embryonic lethality which might be associated with expression in other tissue types. The *lox*/Cre recombinase system also offers the potential for using inducible promoters to introduce the genetic deficiency at any chosen time in the life of the animal.

It should be anticipated that mutant mice of the type described here should become widely and freely available. Support from nonprofit and federal sources has been provided to The Jackson Laboratories to initiate an Induced Mutant Resource to provide for the ready availability of these mutant mice (25). Mutations in CD18, ICAM-1, P-selectin, and many other inflammatory molecules are already available through this mechanism, and it is expected that many or most biologically important mutant animals ultimately will be available through the Induced Mutant Resource or similar facilities.

TESTING DISEASE HYPOTHESES

Mice with mutations such as those already reported for CD18, ICAM-1, P-selectin, and L-selectin and other mice in development are ideally suited for testing the role of these molecules in the pathogenesis of disease models. Our laboratory is generally interested in testing the hypothesis that reduced expression of inflammatory CAMs would reduce the susceptibility to many disease processes which have an inflammatory component. These might include inflammatory bowel disease, asthma, type I diabetes mellitus, various forms of arthritis, autoimmune diseases, and atherosclerosis. Testing of this hypothesis is being initiated using the mutations described to analyze for protection against collagen induced arthritis, experimental autoimmune encephalomyelitis, and atherosclerosis induced by apolipoprotein E deficiency. If mutations in a particular inflammatory CAM protect against a disease process, the results would suggest that pharmacologic approaches to blocking the function or expression of that inflammatory CAM would have therapeutic potential.

ACKNOWLEDGMENTS

We thank Drs. Klaus Ley, Claire Doerschuk and Philip King for critical reading of the manuscript and for sharing unpublished data and Dr. Richard Hynes for providing unpublished manuscripts. This work was supported by NIH grants AI32177 (ALB), and GM15483 (DCB), and AI01102 (ETS) and by the Deutsche Forschungsgemeinscharft (K S-K).

REFERENCES

1.   Butcher EC. Leukocyte-endothelial cell recognition: Three (or more) steps to specificity and diversity. Cell 1991; 67:1033-1036.

2.   Harlan JM, Liu DY. Adhesion: Its Role in Inflammatory Disease. New York: W. H. Freeman and Company, 1992.

3.   Lasky LA. Selectins: Interpreters of cell-specific carbohydrate information during inflammation. Science 1992; 258:964-969.

4.   Springer TA. Traffic signals for lymphocyte recirculation and leukocyte emigration: The multistep paradigm. Cell 1994; 76:301-314.

5.   Albelda SM, Smith CW, Ward PA. Adhesion molecules and inflammatory injury. FASEB J 1994; 8:504-512.

6. Anderson DC, Kishimoto TK, Smith CW. Leukocyte adhesion deficiency and other disorders of leukocyte adherence and motility. In: Scriver CR, Beaudet AL, Sly WS, Valle D, editors. The Metabolic and Molecular Bases of Inherited Disease. 7th ed. New York: McGraw-Hill,Inc. 1994:3955

7. Bradley A. Teratocarcinomas and Embryonic Stem Cells; A Practical Approach. Oxford: IRL Press, 1987.

8. Sedivy JM, Joyner AL. Gene Targeting. New York: W.H.Freeman & Company, 1992.

9. Capecchi M. Altering the genome by homologous recombination. Science 1989; 244:1288-1292.

10. Frohman MA, Martin GR. Cut, paste, and save: New approaches to altering specific genes in mice. Cell 1989; 56:145-147.

11. Wilson RW, Ballantyne CM, Smith CW, Montgomery C, Bradley A, O'Brien WE, et al. Gene targeting yields a CD18-mutant mouse for study of inflammation. J Immunol 1993; 151:1571-1578.

12. Sandberg ET, Sligh JE, Hawkins HK, Rich SS, Beaudet AL. Mutations of cell adhesion molecules CD18 and ICAM-1 impair lymphocyte function in mice. Pediatr Res 1993; 33:157A.

13. Yang JT, Rayburn H, Hynes RO. Embryonic mesodermal defects in $\alpha 5$ integrin-deficient mice. Development 1993; 119:1093-1105.

14. Sligh JE, Ballantyne CM, Rich SS, Hawkins HK, Smith CW, Bradley A, et al. Inflammatory and immune responses are impaired in ICAM-1 deficient mice. Proc Natl Acad Sci U S A 1993; 90:8529-8533.

15. Xu H, Gonzalo JA, St.Pierre Y, Williams IR, Kupper TS, Cotran RS, et al. Leukocytosis and resistance to septic shock in intercellular adhesion molecule 1-deficient mice. J Exp Med 1994; 180:95-109.

16. King PD, Sandberg ET, Selvakumar A, Fang P, Beaudet AL, Dupont B. Tissue distribution and function of novel isoforms of murine ICAM-1 generated by alternative RNA splicing. Blood Suppl 1994; In press.

17. Wolitzky B, Kwee L, Terry R, Kontgen F, Steart C, Rumberger JM, et al. Targeted disruption of the murine E-selectin and VCAM-1 genes. J Cell Biochem Suppl 1994; 18A:300.

18.   Mayadas TN, Johnson RC, Rayburn H, Hynes RO, Wagner DD. Leukocyte rolling and extravasation are severely compromised in P selectin-deficient mice. Cell 1993; 74:541-554.

19.   Arbonés ML, Ord DC, Ley K, Ratech H, Maynard-Curry C, Otten G, et al. Lymphocyte homing and leukocyte rolling and migration are impaired in L-selectin-deficient mice. Immunity 1994; 1:247-260.

20.   Ley K, Bullard D, Arbonés ML, Bosse R, Vestweber D, Tedder TF, et al. Sequential contribution of L- and P-selectin to leukocyte rolling in vivo. J Exp Med 1994;

21.   Hasty P, Ramirez-Solis R, Krumlauf R, Bradley A. Introduction of a subtle mutation into the *Hox*-2.6 locus in embryonic stem cells. Nature 1991; 350:243-246.

22.   Valancius V, Smithies O. Testing an "in-out" targeting procedure for making subtle genomic modifications in mouse embryonic stem cells. Mol Cell Biol 1991; 11:1402-1408.

23.   Smithies O, Kim HS. Targeting gene duplication and disruption for analyzing quantitative genetic traits in mice. Proc Natl Acad Sci USA 1994; 91:3612-3615.

24.   Barinaga M. Knockout mice: Round two. Science 1994; 265:26-28.

25.   Sharp JJ, Davisson MT. The Jackson Laboratory Induced Mutant Resource. Lab Animal 1994; 23:32-40.

AAS 47
Inflammation:
Mechanisms and Therapeutics
© 1995 Birkhäuser Verlag Basel

SITE-DIRECTED MUTAGENESIS - MOLECULAR BIOLOGY AND RATIONAL DRUG DESIGN

G. Ju, E. Labriola-Tompkins, T. Varnell, V. Madison, and B. Graves

Roche Research Center, Hoffmann-La Roche Inc., Nutley, New Jersey, USA

SUMMARY: Using site-directed mutagenesis, we have determined the location and composition of the binding sites in human IL-1α and IL-1β for the Type I IL-1 receptor (IL-1R). The binding site in each ligand is a discontinuous epitope made up of at least seven amino acids whose side chains are exposed on a contiguous region of the protein surface. Although human IL-1α and IL-1β have similar affinities and cross-compete for binding to the human Type I IL-1R, the binding site residues are not identical in the two ligands. In addition, the residues in the binding site of each ligand contribute differently to binding of the human versus the mouse IL-1R. The structure of the IL-1 binding site has implications for the rational design of IL-1 antagonists.

INTRODUCTION

Interleukin 1 (IL-1) is a potent polypeptide hormone that can induce a wide spectrum of immunological and inflammatory activities (1). IL-1α and IL-1β belong to a family of homologous proteins which includes the IL-1 receptor antagonist (IL-1ra). All three IL-1 proteins bind to the Type I IL-1R with the same apparent affinity (K_D = 20-50 pM). In contrast to IL-1α and IL-1β, IL-1ra binds to the IL-1R but has no agonist activity and is therefore a pure antagonist. IL-1α and IL-1β also bind with high affinity to the Type II IL-1R found on B cells, neutrophils, and macrophages.

The biological effects of IL-1 and the observation that IL-1 levels are elevated in inflammatory states such as rheumatoid arthritis (RA), suggest that there would be beneficial effects to antagonizing this proinflammatory cytokine. Protein-based antagonists of IL-1 have been shown to decrease or inhibit inflammatory and autoimmune diseases in animals. Both soluble Type I IL-1R and IL-1ra are in clinical trials for treatment of sepsis, RA, and late-phase cutaneous allergy. Therefore, the rationale for the therapeutic utility of an IL-1 antagonist is well established (2). A small molecule, non-protein IL-1 antagonist would have obvious advantages over the protein-based antagonists currently in development.

To discover such a compound, the novel approach of rational drug design of a receptor antagonist is being pursued. Such an approach ideally requires detailed knowledge of the structure of the ligand and the amino acids that bind to the receptor. The 3-D structures of the IL-1 agonists have been determined (3, 4). We have used the method of site-directed mutagenesis to determine the binding site in IL-1α and IL-1β for the Type I IL-1R (5, 6).

MATERIALS AND METHODS

Plasmids for expression of IL-1α and IL-1β have been described previously (5, 6). Methods for site-directed mutagenesis and competitive binding to Type I and Type II IL-1R's have been described (5, 6).

RESULTS AND DISCUSSION

Using site-directed mutagenesis, we first identified Lys93 and Arg4 in IL-1β as critical for binding to the Type I IL-1R expressed on murine EL-4 cells (5, Table 1). Lys93 and Arg4 were located in one region of the crystal structure of IL-1β (3). When we examined all of the amino acids adjacent to Lys93 and Arg4 in this region, we identified five more residues (Leu6, Phe46, Ile56, Lys103, Glu105) that were critical for receptor binding. In the crystal structure, the side chain of each of these residues was extended and exposed for receptor interaction. Therefore, the binding site in IL-1β for the murine Type I IL-1R is composed of at least seven residues, forming a discontinuous epitope clustered in one region of the ligand (5). The relatively small size of this epitope ($\sim$430 Å^2) is amenable to the design of small molecule antagonists.

For drug design, it was important to determine the residues in IL-1β required for binding to the human Type I IL-1R. Therefore, the IL-1β analogs that showed decreased binding to the murine Type I IL-1R were assayed for binding to the recombinant human Type I IL-1R expressed on CHO cells. We noted both qualitative and quantitative differences in the interaction of IL-1β with the two species of receptors (Table 1). Five of the seven residues remained essential for binding to the human receptor (Arg4, Phe46, Ile56, Lys93, Glu105) while two residues contributed only minimally to receptor binding (Leu6, Lys103). We also determined that substitution of Glu51 (adjacent to Ile56) with Arg caused a significant ($>$10-fold) reduction in competitive binding to the human IL-1R, but had no effect on binding to the mouse receptor. With the exception of Lys 93, the decrease in binding to the human IL-1R noted with each substitution ($\sim$2- to 12-fold) was generally less than the decrease seen with the murine IL-1R ($>$100-fold). Although IL-1β has identical affinities for the human and mouse Type I IL-1R's, these data indicate that there are distinct differences in the interactions of each of the binding residues with each species of receptor.

Table 1. Species-specificity of Type I IL-1 receptor binding residues in IL-1β

IL-1β Analog	Mouse Type I IL-1R[a]	Human Type I IL-1R[b]
Wildtype	100	100
Arg4-Ala	$<$1	8
Leu6-Ala	$<$1	31
Phe46-Ala	$<$1	17
Ile56-Ala	$<$1	14
Lys93-Ala	$<$1	$<$1
Lys103-Ala	$<$1	40-70
Glu105-Ala	$<$1	13-14
Glu51-Arg	100	$<$10

[a] % competitive binding to the natural mouse Type I IL-1R on EL-4 cells.
[b] % competitive binding to the recombinant human Type I IL-1R on CHO cells.

The ideal IL-1 antagonist should inhibit binding of both IL-1 ligands. When we examined the structure of IL-1α (4) in the region homologous to the binding site in IL-1β for the Type I IL-1R, we noted that only three of the seven binding residues were absolutely conserved in both ligands (6). Substitution of two of these three residues (Arg12 and Ile64) caused a significant reduction in binding to the human Type I IL-1R, while substitution of the third conserved residue (Lys96) reduced binding slightly. Substitution of each of the four aligned but non-conserved residues in IL-1α showed that Thr111 and Trp109 were also critical for binding, while Ala substitution of Ile14 and Lys15 resulted in less than 3.5-fold decrease in activity. A double substitution of Asp60Asp61 to AlaAla caused a 50-fold decrease in competitive binding; the Asp residues align with Glu51 in IL-1β. Therefore, although the binding site in IL-1α for the human IL-1R is located in a homologous region to the IL-1β binding domain, its composition is significantly different. Like IL-1β, the IL-1α binding residues also showed variations when comparing their interactions with the mouse and human receptors (6).

In summary, the binding site residues for IL-1R's are not conserved among the IL-1 ligands. Using mutagenesis, we have noted that there are significant and unexpected differences in the binding of specific residues to mouse vs. human Type I IL-1R's, as well as differences between the binding residues in IL-1α and IL-1β for each receptor. These results suggest that, in contrast to their identical binding affinities, each of the ligands has unique molecular interactions with each species of receptor. The information on the binding site residues in the IL-1 ligands is being used for the rational design of potent, small molecule IL-1 antagonists.

REFERENCES

1. Schmidt JA, Tocci M. In: Peptide Growth Factors and Their Receptors I. Sporn MB, Roberts AB, editors. New York: Springer, 1990: 473-521.

2. Dinarello CA. Interleukin-1 and interleukin-1 antagonism. Blood 1991; 77:1627-1652.

3. Priestle JP, Schär H-P, Grütter MG. Crystallographic refinement of interleukin 1β at 2.0 Å resolution. Proc Natl Acad Sci USA 1989; 86: 9667-9671.

4. Graves BJ, Hatada MH, Hendrickson WA, Miller JK, Madison VS, and Satow Y. Structure of interleukin 1α at 2.7 Å resolution. Biochem 1990; 29: 2679-2684.

5. Labriola-Tompkins E, Chandran C, Varnell TA, Madison VS and Ju G. Structure-function analysis of human IL-1α: identification of residues required for binding to the human type I IL-1 receptor. Prot Engin 1993; 6: 535-539.

6. Labriola-Tompkins E, Chandran C, Kaffka KL, Biondi D, Graves BJ, Hatada M, Madison VS, Karas J, Kilian PL, and Ju G. Identification of the discontinuous binding site in human interleukin 1β for the type I interleukin 1 receptor. Proc Natl Acad Sci USA 1991; 88: 11182-11186.

AAS 47
Inflammation:
Mechanisms and Therapeutics
© 1995 Birkhäuser Verlag Basel

C. Gordon Van Arman Scholarship Competition
7th International Conference of the
Inflammation Research Association

J. S. Kerr
The DuPont Merck Pharmaceutical Company, Wilmington, DE 19898-0400

The Inflammation Research Association sponsored a competition to encourage exploratory and applied research in inflammation among graduate students and post-doctoral fellows. Twelve researchers entered the third biennial competition for the C. Gordon Van Arman Awards at the 7th International Conference in White Haven, PA on September 25-29, 1994.

The awards have been named to recognize the example of C. Gordon Van Arman who has had a long and distinguished research career as an industrial scientist during which he published over 100 scientific papers. The development of the drugs diphenoxylate, disopyramide, sulindac, and diflunisal can be directly attributed to his work. In 1970, Dr. Van Arman along with Edward L Takesue, Marvin E. Rosenthale and Mary Lee Graeme founded the Inflammation Research Association as an informal forum for bench scientists to exchange research ideas about inflammatory diseases. By establishing this award, the Inflammation Research Association wishes to encourage young scientists to perform high quality research which focuses on inflammation.

The Scholarship Committee selected the award winners based on a poster presentation to the committee (50%), a mini-paper (25%), and an oral presentation (25%). All finalists' expenses were paid, including registration, room and board, and travel. The prizes of $1,00 (1st), $500 (2nd), $250 (3rd), and $150 (2 honorable mentions) were announced at the Conference Banquet.

The winners were:

1st place: Malinda Longphre, The Johns Hopkins School of Hygiene and Public Health, Baltimore, MD.

2nd place: Karen Ann Ribbons, Louisiana State University Medical Center, New Orleans, LA.

3rd place: Robert E. Smith, University of Michigan Medical School, Ann Arbor, MI.

Honorable Mentions: Maja Stefanovic-Racic, University of Pittsburgh School of Medicine, Pittsburgh, PA., and Dean Willis, St. Bartholomew's Hospital Medical College, London, England.

The Van Arman Award participants added a refreshing and scholarly dimension to the Conference and we are looking forward to future competitions.

Scholarship Committee:
Chairperson: J. S. Kerr
Members: R. P. Carlson   I. G. Otterness
                 R. R. Harris   A. F. Welton
                 L. M. Killar   J. M. Young

The following abstracts are from the winners of the Gordon Van Arman Scholarship Competition:

MAST CELLS CONTRIBUTE TO OZONE-INDUCED NASAL INFLAMMATION AND EPITHELIAL DAMAGE IN MICE

Malinda Longphre

Exposure to the common air pollutant ozone (O_3) produces inflammation and stimulates epithelial proliferation in the airways of humans and animal models. A murine model of mast cell deficiency was employed to test the hypothesis that mast cells are necessary for the initiation of inflammation and epithelial proliferation in the murine nasal airways following O_3 exposure. We exposed mast cell sufficient (+/+), mast cell deficient (W/W^v), and mast cell repleted mice ($BMT/W/W^v$) to 2ppm O_3 or filtered air for 3h. Nasal lavage was performed at two timepoints (6h and 24h recovery) for analysis of differential cell counts and protein content. Epithelial injury and proliferation were determined by light microscopy and bromodeoxyuridine labeling in the nasal epithelium. Relative to air controls, O_3 caused significant increases in inflammatory indicators (NL macrophage number and protein), epithelial damage (NL epithelial cell number and histopathology), and epithelial proliferation (BrdU labeling) in +/+ mice, but little change in W/W^v mice. Mast cell repletion of the W/W^v mice confirmed these results by restoring the inflammatory responses to O_3. These observations are consistent with the hypothesis that mast cells significantly modulate the inflammatory and proliferative responses to O_3 in the murine nasal airways.

NITRIC OXIDE RELEASE AND THE PATHOGENESIS OF CHRONIC IDIOPATHIC COLITIS IN THE RHESUS MONKEY

Karen A. Ribbons

The potential role of nitric oxide (NO) release in the pathogenesis of chronic idiopathic colitis in the rhesus macaque was investigated. Morphological characteristics of the colitis together with the site, enzyme source and magnitude of nitric oxide production were assessed in six juvenile rhesus macaques diagnosed with chronic colitis. Histopathological features of the colitis included a diffuse lymphocytic and plasmocytic infiltration, crypt abscesses, crypt hyperplasia and reduced goblet cell numbers, observed along the entire length of the colon. Systemic NO release was increased in colitic monkeys with nitrate and nitrite levels in plasma and urine of 165 $\pm$ 66μM and 506 $\pm$ 125μM respectively, compared to normal values of 20μM and 91 $\pm$ 29μM respectively. NADPH diaphorase staining was used to localize nitric oxide synthase activity in the colonic tissue. In the normal colon, staining was localized in the neuronal elements of the submucosa and muscularis whereas in the inflamed colon, additional mucosal staining was detected within the crypt abscesses and at the luminal surface. Using RT-PCR, inducible nitric oxide synthase (i-NOS) gene expression was detected in the colonic mucosa from colitic monkeys but was absent in the normal colon. Taken together these results suggest that chronic idiopathic colitis in the rhesus macaque is associated with an increase in nitric oxide release and i-NOS gene expression.

PRODUCTION AND FUNCTION OF MURINE MONOCYTE CHEMOATTRACTANT PROTEIN-1 IN BLEOMYCIN-INDUCED LUNG INJURY

Robert E. Smith

We investigated the role of monocyte chemoattractant protein-1 (MCP-1) in bleomycin-induced lung injury, a model of interstitial lung disease. Bleomycin stimulates a T-cell dependent pulmonary inflammatory response characterized by an increase in leukocyte infiltration, fibroblast proliferation and collagen synthesis. Intratracheal challenge of CBA/J mice with bleomycin resulted in a significant time-dependent increase in MCP-1 protein levels both in whole lung homogenates and broncho-alveolar lavage fluid (BALF). These levels of antigen expression temporally correlate with the accumulation of mononuclear phagocytes in the lung. Interestingly, passive immunization of bleomycin-challenged mice with anti-MCP-1 antibodies significantly reduced pulmonary fibrosis. These experiments establish that MCP-1 protein is expressed in the lungs of bleomycin treated mice and support the notion that leukocyte accumulation and activation are linked to fibrosis.

MODULATION OF CHONDROCYTE PROTEOGLYCAN SYNTHESIS BY ENDOGENOUSLY PRODUCED NITRIC OXIDE

Maja Stefanovic-Racic

Addition of interleukin-1 (IL-1) to fragments of rabbit articular cartilage induced the production of large amounts of nitric oxide (NO), and reduced the incorporation of $^{35}SO_4^{2-}$ into cartilage proteoglycans. Composite agarose polyacrylamide gel electrophoresis confirmed that $^{35}SO_4^{2-}$ was incorporated predominantly into aggrecan, and a faster running band which was probably decorin or biglycan. IL-1 inhibited the synthesis of both of the proteoglycan fractions. Addition of S-nitrosoacetylpenicillamine (SNAP), an organic donor of NO, to resting cultures of chondrocytes also inhibited proteoglycan synthesis. Inhibition of NO biosynthesis by N^G-monomethyl-L-arginine (L-NMA) substantially reversed the inhibitory effect of IL-1 upon aggrecan and biglycan/decorin biosynthesis. L-NMA also increased prostaglandin E_2 (PGE_2) synthesis by IL-1 stimulated chondrocytes, and addition of PGE_2 partially reversed the suppressive effect of IL-1 upon proteoglycan synthesis. These data implicate NO in the mechanism through which IL-1 inhibits proteoglycan synthesis.

EXPRESSION AND MODULATORY EFFECTS OF HEME OXYGENASE IN ACUTE INFLAMMATION IN THE RAT

Dean Willis

Heme oxygenase (HO) is the rate limiting enzyme in the catabolism of heme molecules to the bile pigments which have recently been demonstrated to be strong antioxidants. In this study we analyzed the activity of HO in inflammatory cells isolated from a model of carrageenin induced acute inflammation in the rat. HO activity was significantly higher 24 hours after induction of the inflammation, this increase in activity coincided with the appearance of the highly inducible isoform of HO, Heat Shock Protein 32kDa (HSP32), as detected by Western Blot analysis. Pre-treatment of animals with Tin protoporphyrin, a HO inhibitor, increased cell exudate at 24 hour in this model by 128% as compared to vehicle control. In comparison, pre-treatment with a HO inducer, Ferriprotoporhyrin, decreased inflammatory cell number by 50% and cell exudate by 73% at 24 hours compared to control. These results suggest that HO may represent an endogenous protective mechanism against free radicals in acute inflammation and may be involved in the resolution of acute inflammation. The HSP32 isoform of HO may therefore represent a novel therapeutic target for the modulation of the inflammatory response.

AAS 47
Inflammation:
Mechanisms and Therapeutics
© 1995 Birkhäuser Verlag Basel

NEW ANIMAL MODELS OF INFLAMMATORY DISEASE WORKSHOP

D. S. Grass* and D. E. Griswold**
*DNX Biotherapeutics, Princeton, NJ, USA
**SmithKline Beecham Pharmaceuticals, King of Prussia, PA, USA

Animal models of inflammatory disease are important both as basic research instruments to help elucidate the pathology of various inflammatory conditions and as tools to determine the efficacy of compounds designed to alleviate those conditions. The presentations in this year's workshop were very diverse, but could be categorized into two major groups: those that discussed the characterization of newly developed genetically engineered lines of mice that may become useful models in the future, and those that discussed further characterization and utility of some of the more established classical models of inflammatory disease.

The first three presentations discussed the characterization of three different genetically engineered lines of mice. The two main approaches taken can be called: 1. gene addition, and 2. gene modification. Both are powerful technologies with distinct applications. Gene addition has been used to map cis acting sequences responsible for gene regulation. In addition, and more relevant to animal modeling, gene addition has been used to determine the effects of overexpressing wild type genes and the effects of overexpressing dominant mutations. Gene modification has been used to create both null mutations and structural mutations. These mutations can help determine the role of the "knocked out" gene or the structural mutation during development or in the adult animal. These mutations need not be dominant.

In the first presentation, David Grass (DNX Biotherapeutics) discussed the production and characterization of transgenic mice expressing human extracellular (Type II) phospholipase A2 (PLA2). These mice were produced to create a model for sPLA2 inhibition. The sPLA2 transgenic mice appeared to be normal during the first week after birth, but many of these transgenic lines of mice went on to develop severe alopecia by age 21 days. Hematoxylin and eosin sections performed on tissues taken at 16 or 19 days of age showed epidermal and adnexal hyperplasia in the skin. Despite the expression of sPLA2 in several tissues (liver, skin kidney, and lung by northern analysis; cartilage and bone by immunohistochemical analysis), there was no evidence of inflammation in young mice in any tissue, and only focal inflammation was found in older adult mice. It is possible that levels of expression in various tissues (cartilage, for example) were beneath a threshold level required to trigger inflammation. Further characterization will center on the effect of triggering inflammation by physical manipulation.

Joseph Dinchuk (The DuPont Merck Pharmaceutical Company) discussed mice which were designed to help elucidate the developmental and physiological significance of murine cyclooxygenase 2. The gene modification approach was taken and the strategy was to create a knockout line of mice such that both transcription and translation of the cyclooxygenase 2 gene were disrupted. This was accomplished, with no apparent deleterious effects to mice heterozygous for the mutated allele. However, mice homozygous for the mutated allele had survival rates to weaning that were approximately 25% of the expected value, although no apparent effect on survival through day 10.5 of fetal life occurred. Those homozygous animals that do survive to weaning can be characterized by polydipsia (excessive drinking) and polyuria (excessive urination). Further characterization will be necessary to explain this phenomenon.

A possible murine model of osteoarthritis was discussed by Howard Haimes (OsteoArthritis Sciences, Inc.). Transgenic mice overexpressing the NC4 domain of type IX collagen were produced. Expression of the transgene was driven by the type II collagen promoter. These mice exhibited age related characteristics of osteoarthritis. Knee joint lesions and structural defects in these transgenic mice were similar to those seen in human osteoarthritis. The additional NC4 domains were hypothesized to compete for normal binding sites on type II collagen, thus reducing the mechanical stability of the cartilage.

The second half of the workshop consisted of three presentations describing the utilization of new endpoints to further characterize previously established models. With the use of these new endpoints, the pathophysiology involved in these more traditional models can be better appreciated.

George Stroup (SmithKline Beecham Pharmaceuticals) discussed the application of dual energy x-ray absorptiometry (DXA) to the analysis of bone changes in the adjuvant arthritic rat. Comparing normal rats and adjuvant arthritic rats on the criteria of bone mineral density, bone mineral content, and bone area, it was found that bone mineral losses in the distal tibia could be followed over time by DXA. Quantification of the changes in bone in this model by a means more convenient than histology provides important information which far outstrips the limited utility of paw volume measurements. This technique may be useful to evaluate the efficacy of compounds in the adjuvant arthritic rat model.

Perhaps one of the most clinically relevant models of inflammatory disease is the colitis seen in the Cotton-top tamarin. Neil Clapp (University of Tennessee) presented work in which an LTB4 antagonist, SC-53228 (Searle Research and Development), was administered to these animals. A detailed analysis including colonic biopsy determined these animals to have persistent, active colitis. After 8 weeks of treatment, there was dramatic improvement in these animals, with no or minimally active colitis after treatment. Half of the animals in the study had no active colitis 7 months after treatment, although normally, cotton-top tamarins have recurring colitis after a treatment regimen is stopped. This compound may have a role in the future management of human ulcerative colitis.

In the final presentation, Ivan Otterness (Pfizer, Inc.) discussed attempts to correlate inhibition of locomotor activity and histological changes in cartilage and soft tissue in an IL-1 induced arthritis of the Golden syrian hamster. An acute arthritis was induced by intraarticular injection of IL-1. Although a transient inhibition of spontaneous wheel running was found following the injection of IL-1, the effect did not last longer than one night after the injection. In fact, histologic examination showed the presence of inflammatory cells, soft tissue swelling, and cartilage proteoglycan loss, at the time locomotor activity had been restored to normal. The results suggest that locomotor activity does not correlate with the progression of arthritis in this model. Thus it appears that the IL-1 induced hyperalgesia is independent of synovitis and inflammatory cell infiltration. This model may provide additional information which will contribute to the understanding and study of inflammatory pain associated with the arthritic joint.

AAS 47
Inflammation:
Mechanisms and Therapeutics
© 1995 Birkhäuser Verlag Basel

CELL ADHESION WORKSHOP

J. M. Lackie[1] and A. Aruffo[2]
[1]Yamanouchi Research Institute, Oxford, UK
[2]Bristol-Meyers Squibb, Seattle, WA 98121

7th Inflammation Research Association Meeting: Mountain Laurel, Pennsylvania.
September 25th - 29th, 1994.

It is now generally accepted that the entry of leucocytes into inflammatory lesion depends upon a series of adhesive interactions between leucocytes and endothelial cells and that some of the adhesion molecules may offer targets for novel anti-inflammatory drugs. Initial adhesion from flow depends upon selectins, either on the endothelial cells (E- and P-selectin) or on the leucocyte (L-selectin). Once the leucocyte is stationary a second family of adhesion molecules come into play, the integrins and their ligands, CAMs of various sorts. The differential expression of adhesion molecules on various leucocytes probably plays an important part in determining which cells will infiltrate a lesion. Changes in the expression of adhesion molecules or their ligands with time will also influence the temporal pattern of cellular infiltration at a particular site. The active transmigration of leucocytes across the endothelium depends upon the integrins and defects in $\beta 2$ integrins prevent transmigration in Leucocyte Adhesion Dysfunction (LAD), though not the margination, nor the movement of these deficient cells in a 3-D environment such as connective tissue. Thus these two phases of adhesion are separable in functional, temporal and molecular terms; the selectins being essential for initial trapping but irrelevant for the adhesive interactions involved in endothelial transmigration.

Various strategies for interfering with these adhesive interactions can be visualized, though whether they all offer good therapeutic opportunities remains to be seen. Direct blockade of the adhesion site with site-specific antibody or soluble receptor is the most obvious but least attractive because of the cost involved in producing and delivering the appropriate large molecules. Nevertheless, such blockade provides good evidence for the validity of the particular molecule as a target. Thus the work presented by Simon Blake (Celltech) on the use of anti-E-selectin antibody partially inhibiting TNFα-induced inflammation in baboon skin, and that presented by Anuk Das (National Heart & Lung Institute, London) on the effects of antibodies to VLA4 and CD18 inhibiting eosinophil infiltration into the lungs of guinea pigs are important in that they show that blockade is potentially of therapeutic value. Nevertheless, Das' observation that complete inhibition of cellular infiltration requires that both VLA4 and CD18 are blocked does indicate one of the problems: there is redundancy in the system. Inhibitors that work well in defined *in vitro* systems may be much less effective in the real environment, and inhibiting multiple cell adhesion mechanisms may be necessary for *in vivo* efficacy.

Competitive ligands might offer a better alternative to blocking the adhesion and many hopes have been raised by the idea of small sialylated oligosaccharides as competitive ligands for selectins. RM Campbell (Hoffman LaRoche) presented work on the use of sialyl-Lewis X analogues: although these do inhibit, the results *in vivo* seem rather disappointing, possibly because of their short half-life and lack of selectivity, though there are indications that the endogenous ligand is more complex. By modifying the ligand the structural requirements for binding are becoming clearer and it may be that more potent and longer-lived competitive ligands will be developed.

Since the expression of adhesion molecules changes during the induction of an inflammatory response, another strategy is to inhibit the functional upregulation of selectins or integrins. This approach could involve interference with the inducing cytokine and Marian Nakada (Centocor) showed that antibodies to TNFa would reduce the upregulation of E-selectin, ICAM-1, and VCAM. However, it is also clear from her work that the regulation of adhesion molecule expression is complex and that there is differential regulation of molecules − with the microtubule system of endothelial cells being involved in the clearance of E-selectin but not VCAM-1 from the surface for example. Until the kinetics of adhesion molecule up-regulation and down-regulation are better understood it may be difficult to identify the best targets for intervention. A further complication is that the affinity of integrins can be regulated by intracellular signalling systems, though the way in which this inside-out signalling works is still unknown.

As an alternative to blocking cytokine-induced alterations in adhesion molecule expression, others have looked for inhibitors of other agonists. Peter Will (Hoffman-LaRoche) presented evidence for a PAF antagonist (Ro 24-4736) inhibiting PAF-induced up-regulation of E-selectin on the vasculature in inflamed rabbit skin. Unfortunately the effects seem to be mostly agonist-specific, working only in PAF-induced inflammation, although the PAF antagonist will inhibit a small part (25%) of the response induced by LPS. Certainly blocking the up-regulation of E-selectin by PAF using a PAF-antagonist markedly reduced (94%) the infiltration of labeled neutrophils into PAF-inflamed sites. Susan Uziel-Fusi (CIBA) presented data on inhibition of LTB$_4$-induced up-regulation of CD11b and showed that CGS 25019C would inhibit the ability of human, mouse and monkey neutrophils to upregulate their β2 integrins *ex vivo* in response to LTB$_4$. The utility of these compounds does, of course, depend upon the extent to which a particular inflammatory response is driven by the agonist in question – there have to be some doubts concerning their universal applicability.

A potentially broader-based approach is to interfere with intracellular signalling systems that drive leucocyte activities in inflammation. Robert Smith (Upjohn) presented data on an inhibitor of phospholipase C (U-73122) that had marked effects on adhesion and motility of human neutrophils and that would block the migration of neutrophils across cytokine-stimulated endothelial monolayers in transwell chambers. The same compound also blocks agonist-induced CD11b up-regulation and oxidative burst.

Even from the restricted amount of work that could be covered in a brief workshop session it is obvious that many different approaches are being taken to targeting the adhesion of leucocytes in inflammation and that no single approach yet has a clear advantage.

AAS 47
Inflammation:
Mechanisms and Therapeutics
© 1995 Birkhäuser Verlag Basel

CARTILAGE DEGRADATION AND OSTEOARTHRITIS WORKSHOP

M.J. DiMartino* and E. Mochan**
*SmithKline Beecham Pharmaceuticals, King of Prussia, PA 19406
**Philadelphia College of Osteopathic Medicine, Philadelphia, PA 19131

Matrix Metalloproteinases (MMP), a family of zinc enzymes that includes collagenase, stromelysin and gelatinase, are currently believed to play an important role in cartilage and bone degradation associated with osteo- and rheumatoid-arthritis. It is believed that the induction of these enzymes by cytokines such as IL-1 or TNF leads to an imbalance in the ratio of MMP to endogenous inhibitors (e.g., TIMP). Although numerous *in vitro* inhibitors of MMP have been reported during the past several years, their effectiveness in inhibiting arthritis in animal models has not been firmly established. Thus, there is a need to develop novel inhibitors of MMP or cytokines for the treatment of arthritis. The abstracts presented in this workshop described novel pharmacological, biochemical and immunological approaches to inhibit cartilage or bone degradation in arthritis and included both *in vivo* and *in vitro* studies directed at: 1) interfering with MMP by inhibiting their production, endogenous activation or activity and 2) neutralizing cytokine activity.

The first two presentations described *in vivo* anti-arthritic activities of potent, small molecular weight MMP inhibitors following their oral administration. In studies described by M. DiMartino (SmithKline Beecham), oral administration of hydroxamic acid pseudopeptide MMP inhibitors to adjuvant-induced arthritic rats decreased hindpaw swelling and produced dose related inhibition of bone degradation which was assessed by radiography, dual-energy x-ray absorptiometry and magnetic resonance imaging. During the discussion period, M. DiMartino indicated that examples from this chemical class exhibited stereospecific *in vivo* anti-arthritic activity that correlated with their *in vitro* enzyme inhibitory potency and that their anti-arthritic activity is not due to non-specific anti-inflammatory activity (i.e., inactive in carrageenan-induced rat hindpaw edema) or inhibition of eicosanoid production. However, inhibition of TNF convertase, an activity recently reported for certain examples in this chemical class, cannot be ruled out as a possible anti-arthritic mechanism. In the next presentation, E. O'Byrne (Ciba-Geigy, USA) described oral anti-arthritic activity of CGS 27023A, a non-peptidic sulfonamide based hydroxamic acid inhibitor of MMP in a rabbit osteoarthritis model. CGS 27023A administered daily for eight weeks inhibited proteoglycan and chondrocyte loss in rabbit knees following partial meniscectomy. Synovial hyperplasia and osteophyte formation were moderately increased in rabbits treated with CGS 27023A, suggesting additional effects on connective tissue remodeling.

Inhibition of MMP pro-enzyme activation and synthesis were also presented as potential targets for developing cartilage protectant drugs. E.C. Arner (DuPont Merck) described a unique series of isothiazolones that inhibited IL-1 induced proteoglycan degradation in bovine nasal cartilage by preventing activation of prostomelysin to stromelysin. Evidence was presented to indicate that the compounds bind to cysteine-75 of the pro-enzyme resulting in the production of a less active form of the enzyme. The compounds may also affect activation of other MMP.

E. Mochan (Phila. College of Osteopathic Medicine) presented evidence that Ornithine Decarboxylase (ODC) is involved in MMP mRNA production. IL-1 produced a five-fold increase in ODC mRNA production in human synovial fibroblasts prior to a four-fold increase in MMP mRNA production. Moreover, ODC inhibitors diminished the IL-1 induction of MMP mRNA which could be reversed by the addition of exogenous polyamines. Thus, polyamines appear to be important in the regulation of MMP synthesis. E. Mochan further speculated that inhibition of polyamine biochemical pathways may also be involved in the efficacy of low dose methotrexate.

Wim B van den Berg (University Hospital Nijmegen, The Netherlands) utilized neutralizing antibodies and IL-1ra *in vivo* to investigate the role of TNF and IL-1 in various murine arthritis models. IL-1 production and prolonged message expression were evident in synovial tissue in collagen and Streptococcal cell wall induced arthritis; whereas, TNF expression was more transient and variable. Anti-TNF treatment produced anti-inflammatory activity but limited protection of cartilage damage. In contrast, anti-IL-1 did not produce potent anti-inflammatory activity in certain models but markedly reduced cartilage destruction and prevented proteoglycan synthesis inhibition. These results indicate that IL-1 is a prime target for preventing cartilage destruction.

P. Wooley (Wayne State University School of Medicine, Michigan) described the anti-arthritic effects of CT-112, an octapeptide derived from Platelet Factor 4, in collagen-induced arthritis in mice. Daily subcutaneous administration of CT-112 for ten weeks inhibited the development of arthritis and retarded the progression of established disease. Interestingly, CT-112 did not affect the inflammatory features of arthritis (synovitis and pannus) but decreased the bone erosions and disruption of joint architecture. Thus, CT-112 exhibits a unique anti-arthritic profile. Its mechanism of activity remains to be determined.

In the general discussion period, a debate ensued concerning the utility, appropriateness and necessity of presently used animal models for pre-clinical drug evaluation for osteoarthritis.

One view was that since there are no true models of osteoarthritis and the real test for drug efficacy is in the clinic, the animal models are of little value. On the other side of the debate was the belief that, although there is a need to develop better models, the present animal models provide important information on the pharmacological properties of new anti-arthritic agents and the molecular mechanisms involved in cartilage degradation. Perhaps, at least for the present, a realistic approach would be to combine both viewpoints in drug development - i.e., utilize animal model data for information and direction but do not consider the results essential for a critical path to the clinic.

Overall, the presentations at the workshop supported the hypothesis that cytokines and matrix metalloproteinases are important mediators of cartilage degradation *in vivo* and that inhibitors of these mediators have therapeutic potential for the treatment of osteoarthritis. Moreover, new biochemical and pharmacological approaches for inhibiting cartilage degradation were presented.

AAS 47
Inflammation:
Mechanisms and Therapeutics
© 1995 Birkhäuser Verlag Basel

NEW DRUGS IN PHASE I AND BEYOND WORKSHOP

R. Griffiths* and C. Lanni**
* Pfizer Inc, Groton, CT 06340 and
** Abbott Laboratories, Abbott Park, IL

The aim of the workshop was to encourage an exchange of information on the progress of experimental drugs from the preclinical stage to the early stages of clinical development. Hopefully, some of the drugs discussed will provide improved efficacy in the treatment of a variety of inflammatory diseases. Although an ambitious title because of the commercial sensitivity of this type of data, the organizers were pleased (and relieved) that four of the seven presentations dealt with compounds that actually were in Phase I.

The first presentation by Eric Whalley from Cortech, dealt with the pharmacology of CP-0578 (no, not a Pfizer compound!), which is a dual antagonist of BK_2 and NK_1 receptors. CP-0578 is 15 times more potent as a BK_2 antagonist than an NK_1 antagonist which illustrates one of the major problems in an endeavour such as this, which is to ensure that the intrinsic potency of the compound at two distinct receptors is approximately the same. Many will remember the frustrations involved in trying to achieve dual 5-LO/CO inhibitors with a balanced potency. Importantly, CP-0578 retained activity against human NK_1/BK_2 receptors, and was active in preclinical studies by intravenous infusion.

The next presentation was made by Les Steele from Boots who described the discovery of a series of benzylaminoalkylimidazoles which inhibit cell activation by an as yet unknown mechanism. The lead compound from this series, BTS 71,321, was discovered by screening for inhibitors of arachidonic acid release from zymosan stimulated mouse peritoneal macrophages. Oral activity in models of inflammation and asthma encouraged Boots to progress this compound into human clinical studies. In a single dose, Phase I study, the compound was well tolerated at doses up to 800 mg. Asthma appears to be the initial clinical target for this compound but if the activity in rodents translates into similar activity in humans, then a much broader potential exists for such a compound.

Karen Seibert from Searle presented some very interesting data on progress in the development of inhibitors which are selective for the inducible form of cyclooxygenase (COX-2). This area has progressed very rapidly to the stage where compounds are now entering clinical development. SC-58125, a prototype of this class of compound, inhibits prostaglandin production at sites of inflammation, but not in the gastrointestinal tract. This compound exerts all the anti-inflammatory and analgesic properties of classical cyclooxygenase inhibitors in rodents, without the gastrointestinal side effects. However, it was of interest that a poster at the meeting presented by workers from DuPont Merck described the effects of knocking out the COX-2 gene in mice. The number of mice surviving to 5 weeks of age was only 25% of expected. It will be interesting to see if this finding is predictive of events in longer term toxicology studies with COX-2 inhibitors.

Jim Summers from Abbott introduced the audience to a new PAF receptor antagonist ABT-299. The parent compound is a prodrug which is rapidly converted to the pharmacologically active species. Although a number of PAF antagonists have failed dismally in asthma trials, there is a renewed interest in these agents as treatments for septic shock and associated conditions. The activity of ABT-299 in preclinical models of sepsis was impressive, but then so was IL-1ra and anti-TNF, and we all know what happened to them in clinical trials! Nonetheless, it is to be hoped that ABT-299 and other PAF antagonists fare better than the biotechnology products when they reach the clinic.

The first of two presentations on LTB4 receptor antagonists was made by Don Fretland from Searle. After describing the *in vitro* and *in vivo* credentials of SC-53228, an extremely potent and selective agent, Don then treated the audience to some delightful pictures of the pathology of inflammatory bowel disease (in color too) which were not for the squeamish. This compound was studied in the cotton top tamarin, which spontaneously develops a syndrome similar to human ulcerative colitis. SC-53228 was efficacious by both clinical and biochemical indices and presumably is destined for clinical trials in the human model. Searle are obviously interested in the potential to predict human pharmacokinetics by allometric modeling since pharmacokinetic data for five different species was presented. Improvements in the ability to predict human pharmacokinetics from animal data would be of tremendous value to every drug discovery program.

Kevin Koch from Pfizer then presented preclinical and clinical data on another LTB4 receptor antagonist, CP-105,696. This too is a potent and selective receptor antagonist which shows remarkable efficacy in the murine collagen arthritis model. Clearly it is to be hoped that the efficacy seen with both the Searle and Pfizer compounds in animal models translates into similar efficacy in the clinic. Phase I data on CP-105,696 was presented for the first time. It was well tolerated in a single dose escalation study and, in addition, efficacy was demonstrated using a novel *ex vivo* assay which measures LTB4-induced upregulation of the CD11b molecule on neutrophils. The plasma levels achieved were sufficient to produce a substantial shift in the dose response curve to LTB4 in this assay.

The final presentation was by the Co-Chairman, Carmine Lanni from Abbott, who provided the latest installment in the long-running saga entitled "Can we find a backup to Zileuton?" The latest 5-lipoxygenase inhibitor candidate, ABT-761 is a potent inhibitor with an excellent pharmacokinetic/pharmacodynamic profile in single dose and multi-dose studies in humans. Studies of the rate of glucuronidation in human liver microsomes played a key part in the selection of this compound, since ABT-761 is metabolised 40 times slower than zileuton. This is another example of a drug development program in which the use of drug metabolism studies was fundamental to success.

This workshop highlighted the fact that a number of novel anti-inflammatory agents are approaching the stage at which clinical trials are about to commence. It is to be hoped that these trials will prove successful, and offer clinicians some badly needed new strategies for dealing with the many diseases that have an inflammatory component and which, at the present time, are so poorly treated.

AAS 47
Inflammation:
Mechanisms and Therapeutics
© 1995 Birkhäuser Verlag Basel

LYMPHOCYTE ACTIVATION AND IMMUNOREGULATION WORKSHOP

K. Mollison[1] and F. Dumont[2]
[1]Abbott Laboratories, Abbott Park, IL
[2]Merck, Rahway, NJ

This workshop focused on the pharmacologic inhibition of T lymphocyte activation as an approach towards the development of effective and safe immunosuppressive agents. Triggering of the T cell receptor (TCR)/CD3 complex and of co-stimulatory molecules such as CD28, results in the transcriptional activation of a cohort of immediate/early genes including lymphokine genes, and leads from a quiescent (G0) to a competent (G1) state of the T cells. A second phase involves the response of such competent T cells to secreted lymphokines in an autocrine or paracrine fashion, and drives their entry into the proliferation cycle through G1/S phase progression, with subsequent clonal expansion and acquisition of T cell effector functions. These various steps of the T cell response are amenable to pharmacological intervention for immunosuppressive purpose, as is well illustrated by the six presentations given at the workshop.

The work reported by Kevin Koch and colleagues (Pfizer) exploited the ability of compounds of the FK-506 family of macrocyclic lactones to disrupt the Ca^{2+}/calcineurin-dependent phase of T lymphocyte activation and thereby inhibit lymphokine production. Despite its high potency as an immunosuppressant, the clinical utility of FK-506 (tacrolimus, Prograf^{TM}) is limited by various toxicities, including neurotoxicity and nephrotoxicity. The authors have therefore designed novel analogs of FK-506 with the aim of identifying agents with preserved immunosuppressive activity but reduced toxicity. Their strategy was to introduce carbohydrate residues at the C32 position of the patent-free C21-ethyl analog of FK-506 (FK-520 or ascomycin). The biological characterization of CP-123,369, a rhamno-pyranosyl derivative, was described. Like FK-506, this compound selectively blocks Ca^{2+}-dependent TCR signaling and inhibits IL-2 production, but with a potency approximately 20-fold lower. The compound was orally active in two rodent models of immunosuppressive efficacy (adjuvant arthritis, heterotopic heart transplant), with a potency only 5-10-fold lower than FK-506. However, it was not clear whether the introduced modifications leads to improved oral bioavailability or water solubility as the compound was still administered in cremophor-based vehicle. Most importantly, evaluation of neurotoxicity (aggressive behavior) and of nephrotoxicity (BUN elevation) suggested that CP-123,369 has a greater therapeutic index than FK-506. The authors proposed that the introduced modification may favorably alter the pharmacodynamics of the compound and perhaps decrease its blood-brain barrier penetration. However, no data were presented to support this hypothesis. Although further studies will be needed to explain the relative improvement in therapeutic index of CP-123,369, it appears that agents of this class may prove advantageous for clinical development.

Modulation of the CD28 pathway provides another potential maneuver for immunoregulation. Selective disruption of CD28 signaling may promote antigen specific tolerance. In addition, coapplication of CD3 + CD28 stimuli represents a mode of T cell activation that mimics physiological conditions more faithfully than the standard lectin or Ca^{2+} ionophore + PMA stimulation. This elegant approach has been taken by David Wancio and colleagues (Wyeth-Ayerst) to develop a well-defined *in vitro* model of T cell activation suitable for evaluation of immunosuppressive agents. The activity of various compounds was documented, with rapamycin being the most potent. Cyclosporin A (CsA) was inhibitory in this model, even though, as shown by others, T cell stimulation with anti-CD28 + PMA is resistant to this agent. Presumably, this reflects dependence on a CsA-sensitive component (CD3) for stimulation in the system described here. Compounds that increase cAMP levels such as PDE inhibitors and forskolin inhibited the response. Inhibitors of tyrosine kinases were also active, consistent with the involvement of tyrosine phosphorylation events in both CD3- and CD28-mediated signaling. While proliferation was strongly inhibited, probably as a result of inhibition of IL-2 production, the expression of IL-2R (p55 alpha chain), when it was measured, was less inhibited. It is possible that in these cultures, there is enough residual IL-2 to support IL-2R induction, or that the compounds differentially affect the signaling pathways that lead to IL-2 vs IL-2R transciptional regulation. It was felt that this *in vitro* system should prove useful to identify novel inhibitors of T cell activation.

An original approach for inhibition of IL-2 signal transduction was proposed by Glen Rice and Colleagues from the Cell Therapeutics Inc. group, in collaboration with the laboratories of Mark Jenkins and Barbara Bierer. Earlier studies have shown that IL-2 promotes the hydrolysis of inositol phosphate glycan (GPI) with formation of myristylated phosphatidic acid (mPA) and myristylated diacyl-glycerol (mDAG). The authors have developed an inhibitor (CT-2576), the structure of which was not disclosed (patent pending), but said to be a methyl-xanthine derivative, which alters the IL-2-induced breakdown of GPI such that formation of mPA is inhibited. A functional correlate of this inhibition is the suppression of IL-2-induced proliferation. Compounds like CsA do not have such an effect, and CT-2576 does not inhibit IL-2 production in activated T cells. The production of interferon-gamma was, however, strongly inhibited by CT-2576 and this was shown to reflect a blockade of the autocrine response of T cells to IL-2. Most interestingly, this blockade of IL-2 responsiveness by CT-2576 resulted in induction of antigen-specific energy in several T cells clones. Data were presented indicating that CT-2576 is also immunosuppressive *in vivo*, when administered orally. It is intriguing that CT-2576 was also found to inhibit IL-4 dependent proliferation because earlier studies (Eardley and Koshland) of mDAG formation in the B cell line, BCL-1 have shown that IL-4 exerts a different effect than IL-2, and can actually antagonize IL-2-induced mDAG production as well as proliferation. This suggests that in contrast to B cells, mDAG is not involved in the proliferative signal in T cells. Concern was expressed that CT-2576 might affect other signaling reponses than IL-2 or IL-4, especially insulin signaling, since previous studies have suggested involvement of GPI hydrolysis in this pathway. The authors have not yet examined this possibility.

The immunosuppressive potential of interfering with the secondary phase of T lymphocyte stimulation is best illustrated by the successful use of rapamycin (sirolimus, Rapamune^{TM}) as a potent immunosuppressant. The prospective clinical utility of rapamycin has spurred intense efforts to explore its mechanism of action. Three presentations were devoted to this aspect at the workshop. Rapamycin is known to inhibit the enzymatic activity of the p70 S6 kinase which is involved in the regulation of protein synthesis. Catherine Bansbach and colleagues (Wyeth-Ayerst) therefore examined the effect of rapamycin on protein synthesis, determined by incorporation of ^{3}H-leucine, in mitogenically activated human lymphocytes. While rapamycin did not effect the background level of protein synthesis, it did strongly inhibit the increment induced by activation. Compared to the measurement of ^{3}H-thymidine uptake, the assessment of protein synthesis minimized the donor to donor variability in both the extent of responsiveness and sensitivity to rapamycin inhibition. This parameter of lymphocyte activation may therefore be useful to monitor the *in vivo* immunosuppressive efficacy of the drug.

The primary immunosuppressive effect of rapamycin is believed to result from an inhibition of IL-2-induced T cell proliferation. However, the drug also suppresses the mitogenic action of several cytokines in non-lymphoid cells. Katherine Molnar-Kimber (Wyeth-Ayerst) compared the activity of a series of rapamycin analogs in inhibiting cytokine-dependent and cytokine-independent proliferation in a variety of cell lines. It was found that several analogs do not affect proliferation despite their ability to bind to FKBP12. This indicates that additional properties, other than FKBP binding are required for a pharmacological effect. Moreover, several cell lines were identified which were resistant to the antiproliferative effect of rapamycin This phenotype does not depend on the tissue origin of cells lines. Since rapamycin can be a substrate for the P-glycoprotein involved in multi-drug-resistance, it was suggested that the resistant cells may have acquired increased expression of this protein, which would prevent intracellular accumulation of the drug. This possibility remains to be examined.

The fact that binding to FKBP is not sufficient to account for the antiproliferative action of rapamycin analogs, prompted Katherine Molnar-Kimber, in collaboration with Y. Chen (Columbia University), to search for ternary targets of the rapamycin-FKBP complex. Using a GST-FKBP12 fusion protein, the authors were able to isolate, from lysates for several human lymphoid cell lines, a large MW (210 kDa) protein which was retained only in the presence of immunosuppressive analogs of rapamycin. Amino-acid sequence data as well as partial cloning indicated that this novel protein is identical to the target of rapamycin independently discovered by the groups of Schreiber and Snyder. This protein is also homologous to the targets of rapamycin, TOR1 and TOR2, recently described in yeast. Of interest was the observation that the mammalian protein is found predominantly in the membrane fraction of the cell extracts, although it was not clear whether this fraction represents the plasma membrane or other sub-cellular compartments. This protein, which is postulated to be a lipid kinase due to it partial homology with phosphatidyl-inositol-3 kinase, may mediate at least some of the effects of rapamycin. The existence of additional targets of the FKBP12-rapamycin complex is, however, not excluded and may indeed be suggested by the presence of lower MW bands in the gels. It would appear of great interest to analyze the resistant cell lines mentioned above for expression of these proteins or their interaction with the FKBP12-rapamycin complex. This study was not performed yet. However, it was mentioned that in rapamycin-resistant T cell lymphoma mutants (Dumont et al), evidence was obtained for a loss of interaction of the large MW target (TOR) with the FKBP12-drug complex, further demonstrating the pharmacological relevance of this protein. Continued analysis of the role of this mammalian TOR should help define the mechanisms of cytokine signaling and its inhibition by rapamycin.

AAS 47
Inflammation:
Mechanisms and Therapeutics
© 1995 Birkhäuser Verlag Basel

LIPID MEDIATORS: MECHANISMS

K.B. Glaser* and M.S. Barnette**
*Wyeth-Ayerst Research, Princeton, NY 08543, USA
**SmithKline Beecham, King of Prussia, PA 19406, USA

The mechanisms which regulate lipid mediator production have been an area of intensive research for the past 20 years. Intriguing developments in the areas of phospholipase A_2 (PLA_2) research (inhibitors and regulation) and cyclooxygenase isozymes (regulation of cyclooxygenase-2; COX-2) have generated a renewed enthusiasm for these therapeutic targets. Elucidation of the pathophysiological roles of PLA_2 has been hindered by the lack of specific and orally bioavailable inhibitors of the isoforms of PLA_2 postulated to be involved in arachidonic acid (AA) release, secretory PLA_2 ($sPLA_2$ or 14 kD PLA_2) and cytosolic PLA_2 ($cPLA_2$ or 85 kD PLA_2). The work presented described several new specific inhibitors of PLA_2 (SB 203347 and WAY-125984) with anti-inflammatory properties and new molecular techniques, such as anti-sense DNA, which can be utilized to study the functional role of PLA_2 in intact cells. Another, more classical anti-inflammatory therapeutic approach has been the inhibition of cyclooxygenase, and more recently inhibition of the COX-2 isozyme which may be an important advance toward a "safer" NSAID. Understanding the regulation of the expression of COX-2 is an important facet in the elucidation of the pathophysiological role of the COX-2 isozyme.

L. Marshall (SmithKline Beecham Pharmaceuticals) discussed the properties of SB 203347 (2-[2-[3,5-bis (trifluoromethyl) sulfonamide]-4-trifluoromethylphenoxy] benzoic acid). She presented data indicating that SB 203347 is potent and selective inhibitor of the 14 kD PLA_2 or $sPLA_2$ (IC_{50} =0.5 μM) versus the 85 kD PLA_2 (IC_{50} = 20 μM). Kinetic analysis of the inhibition of 14 kD PLA_2 by SB 203347 indicated a direct interaction with the enzyme. Furthermore, SB 203347 produced a concentration-dependent inhibition of AA release, LTB_4 and PAF formation from A23187 stimulated human neutrophils. Finally, SB 203347 demonstrated topical activity against PMA-induced (ED_{50}s = 0.4-1.3 mg/ear) but not AA-induced ear edema and cellular infiltration. These results demonstrate that selective inhibition of 14 kD PLA_2 or $sPLA_2$ can produce marked anti-inflammatory effects and that the 14 kD PLA_2 is important for the release of AA and the generation of inflammatory mediators.

WAY-125984, a cyclododecyl thiotetronic acid, was described by K. Glaser (Wyeth-Ayerst) as an inhibitor of both sPLA2 and cPLA2 using a ^{3}H-AA labeled *E. coli* system (IC$_{50}$s = 1.5 and 15 µM, respectively). Elucidation of the WAY-125984 structure was accomplished by molecular modeling with a model of human synovial PLA2 using the tetronic acid series of PLA2 inhibitors. Grid calculations of the active site region with a methylene probe (hydrophobic interactions) were utilized to optimize the cyclododecyl group as the best hydrophobic moiety for this series. The thiotetronic acid series was further optimized in cellular assays. WAY-125984 inhibited lipid mediator release in murine resident macrophages (IC$_{50}$s = 0.08 and 0.12 µM for PGE$_2$ and LTC$_4$, respectively, and human neutrophils (IC$_{50}$s of 3.0 µM for both LTB$_4$ and PAF production). Inhibition of AA release (GC mass measurements and [^{3}H]-AA release) was also observed in the murine macrophage (IC$_{50}$s = 2.0 and 4.0 µM, respectively, in the presence of fatty acid free BSA). WAY-125984 demonstrated both topical and oral activity in the TPA ear edema assay (ED$_{50}$s of 90 µg/ear and 100 mg/kg, respectively). Also, beneficial effects were observed in the LPS-induced hypothermia in mice after subcutaneous administration and in preventing adjuvant-induced edema in rats after oral administration. Finally, WAY-125984 (37.5 mg/kg; p.o.; b.i.d.) reduced by 60-80% the incidence and clinical severity of collagen-induced arthritis in mice. These findings show that WAY-125984 is a prototypical orally active PLA2 inhibitor with *in vivo* anti-inflammatory activity in animal models of inflammation. Thus, these two presentations demonstrate that it is possible to design novel selective PLA2 inhibitors and that these inhibitors produce anti-inflammatory effects.

M. Withnall (Rhone Poulonc Rorer) described the differential regulation of sPLA2 and cPLA2 and AA release in alveolar macrophages (AM) and U937 cells using inhibitors of sPLA2 (scalaradial), cPLA2 (arachidonyl trifluromethylketone, AACOCF3) and PKC (Ro-31-8425). In U937 cells but not AMs, PMA enhanced and Ro-31-8425 inhibited [^{3}H]-AA release demonstrating a role for PKC activation in U937 cells. The role of cPLA2 in [^{3}H]-AA release was inferred as reported cPLA2 inhibition by AACOCF3 prevented AA release whereas heparin which binds sPLA2 did not. In support of this finding, published results obtained with scalaradial in AM were also presented. Thus in U937 cells, PKC appeared to be directly involved in [^{3}H]-AA release through cPLA2 via direct phosphorylation or through phosphorylation and activation of MAP kinase which subsequently activates PLA2. These results demonstrate that the mechanism governing [^{3}H]-AA release differs between cell types and stimulants used, and must be considered when interpreting the role of PLA2s in [^{3}H]-AA release.

To investigate the differences between AA release as measured by GC (mass) or radiolabelled AA ([^{3}H]-AA), A. Hoffman (Boehringer Ingelheim) examined the ability of BIRM-270 to inhibit AA release. BIRM-270 is a unique inhibitor of mediator release whose exact molecular mechanism is unknown. However, BIRM-270 is able to inhibit the secretion of $sPLA_2$ and this ultimately leads to an inhibition of AA release. In human neutrophils the difference in methods used to measure AA release was evaluated with BIRM-270. When AA release was measured at either $28\,^\circ C$ or $37\,^\circ C$ it was apparent the $[^3H]$-AA release was identical at both temperatures whereas GC AA release was lower at $28\,^\circ C$. Increasing the temperature from $28\,^\circ C$ to $37\,^\circ C$ decreased the time to peak release from approximately 4 to 2 min. At both $28\,^\circ C$ and $37\,^\circ C$ BIRM-270 produced a greater inhibition of AA release when measured by GC rather than $[^3H]$-AA release. The leftward shift in the dose-response curve for BIRM-270 when measured by GC (mass) may suggest that data from $[^3H]$-AA release may not be reflective of actual AA release within cells and the use of $[^3H]$-AA release may underestimate the effectiveness of inhibitors on AA release. BIRM-270 represents a novel class of lipid mediator modulators useful in the elucidation of the mechanisms of AA release in cells.

Finally, two speakers discussed alternative approaches for investigating the role of lipid mediator formation in inflammation. A. Roshak (SmithKline Beecham Pharmaceuticals) presented an elegant study examining the role of 85 kD PLA_2 or $cPLA_2$ in prostaglandin formation in human monocytes. LPS treatment of monocytes produced an increase in the release of PGE_2 that coincided with a 2 fold increase in the expression of the 85 kD PLA_2 as well as an increase in COX-2 expression. However no change occurred in the amount of the 14 kD PLA_2 ($sPLA_2$) nor did LPS treatment increase its release. Since cycloheximide pretreatment prevented the LPS-induced increase in 85 kD activity, the ability of antisense specific for the 85 kD protein to prevent both the LPS-induced upregulation of this protein as well as the increase in PGE_2 production was examined. Antisense to $cPLA_2$ (85 kD PLA_2) decreased both the activity and protein of this enzyme without altering these levels of COX-2 or the 14 kD form of PLA_2. More importantly, antisense treatment decreased the LPS-induced PGE_2 formation in these cells. These results demonstrate the importance of the 85 kD form of PLA_2 in providing arachidonic acid for the cyclooxygenase pathway in the monocyte.

An alternative approach was discussed by J. Lee (SmithKline Beecham Pharmaceuticals) examining the translation regulation of COX-2 expression in human monocytes. He presented evidence that the SB CSAID^{TM} compounds inhibited the LPS-induced increase in COX-2 protein without altering the steady state mRNA levels. His results suggest a mechanism of action distinct from that of glucocorticoids, namely one of translational repression. Also these compounds did not change the constitutive expression of COX-1. Dr. Lee presented a hypothesis to explain this effect by noting the presence of AU rich regions in the 3' untranslated regions of the mRNA for COX-2 and not COX-1. Since these regions have been implicated in the translation regulation of protein expression for certain cytokines, they may also confer this regulation on COX-2.

This brief summary of the work presented illustrates the exciting new avenues available for the study of lipid mediators in inflammation.

AAS 47
Inflammation:
Mechanisms and Therapeutics
© 1995 Birkhäuser Verlag Basel

INFLAMMATORY CYTOKINES WORKSHOP

B.E. Miller* and E. O'Byrne**
*Sterling Winthrop Inc., Collegeville, PA
**Ciba, Summit, NJ

The workshop opened with an overview of cytokines in inflammation by Dr. Bruce Miller. It was emphasized that, although the cytokine network is complex, our understanding of the role of numerous cytokines in inflammatory diseases is continually expanding. The workshop presentations covered modulation of cytokine production and function and *in vivo* effects of cytokine inhibition.

A pharmacological approach to regulating production of the inflammatory cytokine IL-1β is to inhibit IL-1β converting enzyme (ICE). Dr. Joanne Ohl (Sterling Winthrop, Collegeville, PA) discussed studies on the optimization of IL-1β secretion by cultured human monocytes and inhibition of IL-1β secretion by ICE inhibitors. After activation, cultured monocytes produced both the 31 kD precursor and the 17 kD active, mature IL-1β. The relative proportion of each was dependent on the stimulus for activation. After activation with lipopolysaccharide (LPS), >90% of the total IL-1β secreted was proIL-1β; whereas following activation with *S. aureus*, >80% of the secreted IL-1β was the mature form. ICE inhibitors like WIN 67694 selectively inhibited the release of mature IL-1β from *S. aureus* activated monocytes with no effect on the production or secretion of proIL-1β. In related studies, B.E. Miller, *et al.* (Sterling Winthrop) showed that WIN 67694 also selectively inhibited the release of IL-1β *in vivo* in a murine subcutaneous tissue chamber model. Dr. Alexander MacKenzie (Sandoz, Berne) reported that the ICE inhibitor, SDZ 220-796, reduced paw swelling in the carrageenan-induced rat paw edema model and also reduced LPS-induced fever in rats when administered orally. Together, these studies indicate the potential utility of ICE inhibitors to treat diseases with components of inflammation.

Two papers examined the effects of TNF-α inhibition *in vivo*. Dr. Donald Griswold (SmithKline Beecham, King of Prussia, PA) reported on TNF-α production during the inflammatory response to ultraviolet B (UVB) irradiation in the mouse ear. Mice were exposed to UVB for 30 minutes and TNF-α, myeloperoxidase (MPO), and ear thickness were measured 72 hours later. Administration of a phosphodiesterase inhibitor, rolipram (10 mg/kg, p.o.), inhibited release of TNF-α and MPO and reduced ear swelling suggesting that regulating TNF-α production through modulation of cAMP levels is anti-inflammatory. In contrast, the cyclooxygenase inhibitor naproxen (20 mg/kg, p.o.) enhanced TNF-α production and ear swelling. Dr. Edward Shatzen (Amgen, Thousand Oaks, CA) described the regulation of TNF-α production by CAP 18 peptide, a 32 amino acid C-terminal peptide of a cationic 18 kD protein originally isolated from rabbit granulocytes. CAP 18 peptide inhibits LPS-induced release of TNF-α in human blood with an IC_{50} of 40 nM. *In vivo*, CAP 18 peptide at 0.5 mg/kg, i.p. prevented lethality in *E. coli*-induced peritonitis and LPS-galactosamine endotoxemia. In a poster presentation, Salter and Pettipher (Pfizer, Groton, CT) presented an *in vivo* model for measuring TNF-α in an arthritic joint. Following intra-articular injection of zymosan into rat knees, peak levels of TNF-α were detected in a synovial lavage at 1-2 hours and had declined by 5 hours.

Dr. Sussan Nourshargh and colleagues (Nat'l. Heart Lung Institute, London) studies recruitment of eosinophils in rat skin in response to IL-1 using intravital microscopy. Coadministration of IL-1 with the IL-1 receptor antagonist (IL-1ra) or actinomycin D inhibited cell accumulation demonstrating that the response is receptor mediated and dependent on local protein biosynthesis. The response was also suppressed by i.v. treatment with the PAF antagonist UK-74,505 or an anti-human IL-8 mAb (DM/C7) providing evidence for the involvement of PAF and IL-8 like molecules in the eosinophil accumulation induced by IL-1. This study also provides evidence for IL-8 and/or IL-8-related molecule in the rat, an observation which has not been reported previously.

The role of IL-1 and TNF-α in flares of antigen-induced arthritis was investigated by Dr. A.A.J. van de Loo and coworkers (Nijmegen, The Netherlands). Intra-articular injection of priming antigen induces a flare of inflammation and rapid loss of proteoglycan. Treatment with anti-IL-1(α+β) or IL-1ra before flare induction reduced the inflammatory response and cartilage proteoglycan loss. Neutralizing antibody to TNF-α had no effect. Cartilage degradation in response to injection of IL-1 was enhanced in knees of arthritic mice compared to naive joints suggesting that chondrocytes in arthritic cartilage are primed to respond to IL-1. Ongoing studies are investigating chondrocyte IL-1 receptor expression.

An interesting finding, reported by Dr. Nicolas Hall (Bath, UK), is that mononuclear cells (MNC) from rheumatoid arthritis patients express markedly impaired ouabain-sensitive Na^+/K^+ ATPase sodium pump activity. In normal MNC, ouabain induces transcription of IL-1β mRNA and suppresses IL-6 production. This pattern of cytokine production, IL-1 induction/IL-6 suppression, is also observed when MNC are incubated with the sodium ionophore monensin. These observations suggest that downregulation of Na^+/K^+ ATPase activity on rheumatoid MNC may predispose these cells to produce increased quantities of IL-1β and suggests a potential mechanism to account for the over-production of IL-1 and resulting tissue injury in rheumatoid joints.

The presentations at the workshop demonstrate that progress is being made in approaches to evaluate the downstream effects of inhibiting cytokine activity. In the near term, the models reported here and others should further our understanding of the role of individual cytokines in the development and progression of the inflammatory response.

AAS 47
Inflammation:
Mechanisms and Therapeutics
© 1995 Birkhäuser Verlag Basel

PULMONARY INFLAMMATION WORKSHOP

A.N. Payne* and W. Selig**
* Wellcome Research Laboratories, Beckenham, Kent, BR3 3BS, England
**Cortech, Denver, CO 80221, USA

Pulmonary inflammation is now recognised to be a fundamental feature of asthma and other pulmonary diseases such as bronchitis. As such, increased understanding of this process is a key issue in the search for new and more effective therapeutics for the control of lung disease. In asthma, eosinophils, neutrophils, mast cells, lymphocytes are all thought to be involved, in conjunction with a cocktail of soluble mediators, e.g. histamine, leukotrienes, tachykinins, platelet activating factor, cytokines. Many animal models, in particular guinea-pigs, have been used in an attempt to tease apart the relationships between these different cell types and mediators. While it is appreciated that these models may be imperfect analogues of the clinical situation, they do offer the opportunity of investigating certain facets of the inflammatory process, which may translate across to man.

In the first presentation, Dr. M. Yeadon (Wellcome Research Laboratories, Beckenham, UK) described the differential modulation by betamethasone of allergen-induced early neutrophilia and late eosinophilia in the lungs of actively sensitised guinea-pigs. The aim of this investigation was to characterise more precisely the allergic inflammatory response following challenge with inhaled allergen (ovalbumin) and the anti-inflammatory effect of this steroid. Allergen inhalation selectively increased tissue myeloperoxidase (MPO) activity and the number of neutrophils in bronchoalveolar lavage (BAL) samples at 1h, but not at subsequent time points. These increases were accompanied by a concomitant reduction in MPO/BAL neutrophil. By 8h, and for a further 64h later, the number of eosinophils in the BAL were elevated as well as tissue eosinophil peroxidase (EPO). The EPO/BAL eosinophil was also increased. Betamethasone (1-5 mg/kg p.o.) given 18h and 2h prior to allergen challenge blocked the early accumulation of neutrophils in the BAL as well as the rise in tissue MPO. It did not however block the fall in MPO/BAL neutrophil. When given 1h pre and 12h post challenge, betamethasone blocked the late accumulation of eosinophils in the BAL, and the rise in tissue EPO but increased further EPO/BAL eosinophil. Hence while betamethasone inhibited recruitment of both eosinophilia and neutrophils in the BAL and lung tissue, it had differential effects on the cell peroxidase levels. This may be explained by the inhibition by this steroid of eosinophil, but not neutrophil, degranulation. In subsequent discussion, numerous points were raised, including the desirability of checking whether betamethasone was an inhibitor of BAL peroxidase and whether or not it influenced pulmonary hyperaemia following allergen challenge. It also had to be borne in mind that elevation of peroxidase activity did not necessarily equate to tissue damage.

The next presentation was given by Dr. R. Howell (Wyeth-Ayerst Research, Princeton, NJ, USA). He described the pulmonary anti-allergic and antiinflammatory effects of a novel, orally-active phosphodiesterase IV inhibitor (WAY-127093B; (S)-3-[cyclopentyloxy-4-methoxyphenyl] -2- methyl -5- oxo -N- (3-pyridinyl methyl) -1-pyrazolidine carboxamide maleate salt) in guinea-pigs and rats. This compound had an IC_{50} of 9 nM versus canine tracheal PDE IV *in vitro*. It had an oral ED_{50} of 4.8 mg/kg for inhibition of inhaled allergen (ovalbumin) induced bronchoconstriction in anaesthetised guinea-pigs. This compared with 0.5 mg/kg for rolipram and 44 mg/kg for aminophylline. All three compounds were equally efficacious (73-85% inhibition) versus allergen-induced bronchoconstriction. However, whereas aminophylline was equally effective versus histamine-induced bronchoconstriction, WAY-127093B and rolipram produced much less inhibition. This observation suggested that the latter two inhibitors exerted their effect versus antigen challenge primarily through inhibiting mediator release rather than causing bronchodilation. This is supported by the finding that in guinea-pigs pre-treated with pyrilamine, WAY-127093B (10 mg/kg p.o.) inhibited allergen-induced "leukotriene-dependent" bronchoconstriction to a similar degree as the Abbott 5-LO inhibitor A-78773 given at the same dose. WAY-127093B (ED_{50} 0.3 mg/kg) was more potent than rolipram (ED50 10 mg/kg) in inhibiting antigen-induced accumulation of eosinophils in BAL samples from guinea-pigs. WAY-127093B was also effective in inhibiting antigen-induced BAL eosinophilia and neutrophilia in Brown Norway rats. The compound is now in Phase I clinical trials. In response to questions from the floor, Dr. Howell said that as yet there was no evidence of behavioural side effects or emesis with the compound. No anti-inflammatory investigations had so far been carried out with chronic dosing, hence there was no evidence for tachyphylaxis. The compound also inhibited LPS-induced neutrophilia in rats, whereas rolipram was much less effective in this model.

In the following presentation, Dr. W. Selig (Cortech, Denver, CO, USA) described the effects of two peptidic bradykinin$_2$-receptor antagonists, CP-0597 (D-Arg^0 [Hyp^3, Thi^5, D-Tic^7, N-Chg^8]BK and Hoe 140 (D-Arg^0 [Hyp^3, Thi^5, D-Tic^7, Oic^8] BK on allergen-induced airway hyperreactivity and bronchoalveolar lavage fluid (BALF) eosinophilia in actively sensitised guinea-pigs. In anaesthetised guinea-pigs, both compounds appeared to be effective antagonists of bradykinin-induced increases in lung resistance, with approximate ID_{50}s of 0.7 and 0.1 ug/kg/min i.v. respectively. They also were effective in inhibiting bradykinin-induced plasma extravasation (ID_{50}s of 2.0 and 0.6 ug/kg/min). Both CP-0597 and Hoe 140 were tested in a model of pulmonary anaphylaxis characterised by enhanced airway reactivity to intravenous bradykinin and BALF eosinophilia (both elevated approximately 5-fold versus controls) at 24h following antigen (ovalbumin) challenge. When administered as either an aerosol (0.1%) 15 min before antigen challenge or intravenously (0.3 and 1.0 ug/kg/min immediately prior to measuring airway hyperreactivity, both compounds inhibited antigen-induced airway hyperreactivity (24h post challenge) to i.v. bradykinin to varying degrees. These findings suggested that antigen-induced airway hyperreactivity to i.v. bradykinin was predominantly mediated through a bradykinin$_2$-receptor. CP-0597 was also shown to be an effective inhibitor of antigen-induced BALF eosinophilia when given as an aerosol (0.01-0.1%) prior to antigen exposure. In contrast, aerosolised Hoe 140 (0.03-0.1%) was ineffective against the elevation of BALF eosinophilia suggesting an as yet unexplained disparity between these two peptidic bradykinin$_2$-receptor antagonists. Dr. Selig ended his presentation by inferring that potent bradykinin$_2$-receptor antagonists such as CP-0597, when linked to other receptor antagonists to form a single drug moiety or heterodimer (a concept currently being explored at Cortech), may be potentially useful therapeutic approaches in treating pulmonary diseases such as asthma. In response to questions from the floor, Dr. Selig said that the relative contribution of oedema to antigen-airway hyperreactivity in the model was uncertain, but the compounds might act to some degree by reducing extravasation. Studies to see whether CP-0597 and/or Hoe 140 similarly inhibited antigen-induced airway hyperreactivity to acetylcholine had not been carried out.

The next speaker was Dr. L. Renzetti (Hoffmann-La Roche, Nutley, NJ, USA). He presented pre-clinical data pertaining to the anti-inflammatory activity of a novel, long acting, VIP receptor agonist, Ro 25-1553, in various allergic and non-allergic guinea-pig models. Aerosolised Ro 25-1553 (0.1%) was shown to effectively inhibit antigen-, vagally-, and bradykinin-induced airway plasma extravasation measured 10 min later. Aerosolised Ro 25-1553 (0.001-0.1%) also dose-dependently inhibited antigen-induced airway hyperreactivity to intravenous substance P and BALF leukocyte (eosinophil and neutrophil) influx 6h after challenge. This effect appeared to be unrelated to the bronchodilator activity of Ro 25-1553 as illustrated by the inability of this VIP analogue (0.1% aerosolised) to inhibit substance-P induced bronchoconstriction at 6h. Intrapulmonary arterial injection of Ro 25-1553 (3-300 µg) dose-dependently inhibited antigen-induced venous effluent histamine release in perfused guinea-pig lungs. As such, Ro 25-1553 may be a novel therapeutic with anti-inflammatory actions useful in the treatment of asthma. Subsequent discussion centered around why VIP itself does not work in some of these assays (instability?) and what contribution (probably little) the secondary release of nitric oxide by VIP had.

Currently there is considerable debate regarding the relative roles of peptido and non-peptido leukotrienes (LTs) in provoking lung inflammation and thus the prospective therapeutic effect of LTD_4 antagonists versus 5-lipoxygenase inhibitors. Dr. D. Underwood (Smith Kline Beecham, King of Prussia, PA, USA) described the results from a study carried out in conscious guinea-pigs in order to characterise more fully the pharmacology of LTD_4- induced bronchoconstriction and eosinophilia. Aerosols of 0.3-30 μg/ml LTD_4, 1 min, caused maximum falls in specific airway conductance (sGaw) of 70-90% at all concentrations tested. BAL measurements and histological studies showed that the bronchoconstrictor effect of inhaled LTD_4 was followed 8-24 hr later by a concentration-related accumulation of eosinophils (3.2-14.5 x baseline) in the bronchial epithelium and sub-epithelium. Neither the bronchoconstrictor, nor the inflammatory effect of inhaled LTD_4 was blocked by cyclooxygenase inhibition using meclofenamic acid. In contrast the LTD_4 antagonist pranlukast (20 mg/kg i.g.) inhibited both effects of LTD_4. On the other hand, the PDE IV inhibitor rolipram (3 & 10 mg/kg i.g.) inhibited LTD_4-induced eosinophilia but had no effect on bronchoconstriction. Other LTD_4 antagonists had also been shown to be effective in this animal model. These results suggest, but do not prove, that LTD_4 antagonists may have an antiinflammatory as well as an anti-bronchoconstrictor effect in asthma.

Dr. P. Sirois (Univ. Sherbrooke, Montreal, P.Q. Canada) described the effect of non-glucocorticoid 21 aminosteroids (lazaroids) on Sephadex bead-induced eosinophilia and bronchial hyperresponsiveness in guinea-pigs. Pretreatment with U-75412E, (1 mg/kg i.p.) for 6 days inhibited both blood and BAL eosinophilia induced by i.v. injection of a sterile suspension of 24 mg G-50 Sephadex beads. Curiously however, a 10-fold higher dose of this compound administered by the same protocol was without effect. Compound U-83836E was also ineffective, but dexamethasone (10 mg/kg) reduced strongly both BAL and blood eosinophilia. The effect of these compounds on Sephadex-induced bronchial hyperreactivity (BHR) was investigated using isolated lower bronchus preparations from animals treated as above. U-75412E at 10 mg/kg i.p. x 6 days, but not at 1 mg/kg, reduced Sephadex-induced BHR to histamine and acetylcholine by approximately 50%. At the same dose, U-83836E also reduced BHR, but to a slightly lesser degree. However dexamethasone was without effect on Sephadex-induced BHR. The data illustrated the complexities of both the Sephadex model and the effects (e.g., bell-shaped dose response curve for U-75412E) of the lazaroid type compounds.

Although there have been many animal studies of the bronchoconstrictor effect of the vascular endothelial cell-derived peptide endothelin-1 (ET-1), there have been few studies of its possible pro-inflammatory effect. In the penultimate presentation, Dr. J. Filep (Maisonneuve-Rosemont Hospital, Montreal, Canada) described how in anaesthetised guinea-pigs, bolus i.v.

injection of ET-1 (0.1-1 nmol/kg) caused dose-related increases in mean arterial blood pressure, hemoconcentration and enhanced albumin extravasation in the trachea and bronchi, but not in the parenchyma. These effects were inhibited substantially, although not totally, by the selective ET_A receptor antagonist FR139317 ((R)2-[(R)-2-1-(hexahydro-1H-azepynil)] carbonyl] amino-4-methylpentanoyl]-3-[3-(1-methyl-1H-indoyl)]propionyl]amino-3-(2-pyridyl) propionic acid) at 2.5 mg/kg i.v. ET-1 also produced a dose-dependent systemic neutropenia (inhibited by either FR139317 or norepinephrine) but did not initiate a influx of neutrophils into the lung tissue. Interestingly ET-1 (10^{-10}-10^{-6}M) did not in itself activate alveolar macrophages *in vitro*, but did potentiate PAF and FMLP-induced superoxide release from these cells. Thus as well as having direct effects on airway and vascular smooth muscle, ET-1 may play a role in the underlying inflammation of asthma. However, confirmation of this must await clinical trials with selective ET_A and ET_B receptor antagonists. Furthermore, it was pointed out during the discussion of this paper that some of the pro-inflammatory effects of ET-1 may be due to the release of secondary mediators such as cyclooxygenase products.

The last presentation of the workshop was by Dr. M. Janusz (Marion Merrell Dow, Cincinnati, OH, USA). He described the pharmacology and pharmacokinetics of selected representatives of a novel series of orally active peptide inhibitors of human neutrophil elastase (HNE). HNE is a serine protease which has been implicated in the destructive processes of a number of chronic inflammatory diseases, not only of the lung, but of other organs too. MDL 101,146, MDL 102,111, MDL 102,823 and MDL 100,948 are 4-(4-morpholinylcarbonyl)-benzoyl], N-(4-morpholinylcarbonyl], N-[(tetrahydro-2H-pyran-4-yl) carbonyl] and N-[2-(4-morpholinyl)ethanoyl]-val-pro-val-pentafluoroethylketones, respectively. While the K_is of these compounds varied considerably (25-170 nM) *in vitro*, *in vivo* they had similar ED_{50}s (15-30 mg/kg) after oral administration in a hamster model of HNE-induced haemorrhage. They were also effective at inhibiting HNE-induced pulmonary haemorrhage in rats. Their $t_{1/2}$ was of the order of 2-4h and was related both to absorption and metabolism which explained their similar *in vivo* (but different *in vitro*) potencies. One of the compounds, MDL 101,146 is currently targeted towards clinical trials in bronchitics.

In summary, as evidenced by the workshop content, the search for new and more efficacious drugs for the treatment of pulmonary inflammation has entered an exciting phase with the advent of clinical trials (either ongoing or imminent) with various differing classes of putative anti-inflammatory agents. At the same time, basic research continues to shed light on the complexities of the inflammatory process and as a corollary will doubtless also suggest possible new targets for therapeutic intervention.

AAS 47
Inflammation:
Mechanisms and Therapeutics
© 1995 Birkhäuser Verlag Basel

NITRIC OXIDE POSTER DISCUSSION

M.J.S. Miller* and N.K. Boughton-Smith**
*Louisiana State University Medical Center New Orleans, LA 70112, USA
**Fisons plc, Loughborough, LEICS LE11 ORH, UK

Nitric oxide (NO) is widely recognized as a potential contributor to inflammation; however, there remains considerable controversy as to its role (pro- or anti-inflammatory), source (cellular and enzyme) and regulation of production (basal vs. inflammation) in various inflammatory processes. A poster discussion group addressed the current controversies surrounding these and other aspects of NO research. The session concluded with a soul-searching evaluation of the potential for specific inhibitors of the inducible isoform of nitric oxide synthase (iNOS) as anti-inflammatory agents.

Nitric oxide can display a host of anti-inflammatory properties, usually defined in acute protocols when the constitutive isoforms of NOS are responsible for NO synthesis. These beneficial effects are largely mediated by activating guanylyl cyclase and raising intracellular cGMP levels. In vascular smooth muscle this leads to vasodilation, in platelets and leukocytes this mechanism prevents adherence to the endothelium. Two abstracts in this session focused on these vascular actions of NO. J. Filep (University of Montreal) discussed the ability of the NOS inhibitor L-NAME, to increase vascular permeability *in vivo*, as determined by Evans Blue dye-bound albumin leakage, under basal conditions. L-NAME was able to potentiate the effects of platelet activating factor or endothelin on vascular permeability. These effects appear to be independent of pressure but may result from actions on leukocyte adhesion. The enzyme source under these acute, basal conditions is likely to be constitutive NOS. However, in studies by Boughton-Smith and Ghelani contrasting conclusions were drawn in a model that results in iNOS expression, *viz*., zymosan peritonitis. Zymosan results in cellular infiltration into the peritoneum, increased vascular permeability and a dramatic increase in local NO production through calcium-independent processes, i.e., iNOS. Increased NO production can be prevented by pretreatment with a NOS inhibitor, L-NAME, or glucocorticoids. These agents attenuate the permeability response independent of changes in leukocyte numbers. NO may be contributing to the increased vascular permeability at numerous levels: as a result of vasodilation or via endothelial injury. However, NO mechanisms alone are not responsible for plasma leakage in this model but its actions bear similarities to actions described for prostaglandins. Additionally, these studies draw attention to the contrasting effects of NO in a manner that is dependent on the enzyme source. A constant theme in the literature is that anti-inflammatory actions of NO are mediated by constitutive isoforms of NOS whereas NO produced from iNOS displays pro-inflammatory characteristics.

An exception to the role of iNOS in inflammation appears to be the chondrocyte, as reported by A.C. Hanglow (Hoffman-LaRoche). IL-1β stimulated cartilage explants degrade their proteoglycan matrix. However, NO appears to attenuate this process, possibly via a matrix metalloproteinase dependent pathway, as the rate of proteoglycan degradation was enhanced by the NOS inhibitor, L-NMA. In the Gordon Van Arman competition M. Stefanoic-Racic in a similar model in rabbits, demonstrated that IL-1 stimulated NO production from cartilage explants were responsible for inhibiting proteoglycan synthesis. In arthritic states, the role of chondrocyte-derived versus synovium-derived NO may differ. In models of arthritis NOS inhibition appears to ameliorate the disease process. J. Selph (Wellcome) demonstrated that the streptococcal cell (SCW) model of arthritis dramatically increased NO synthesis in a manner that parallels the time-course of the model. SCW-induced arthritis is characterized by an initial inflammatory response (1-7 days) with a partial resolution of symptoms followed by a chronic inflammatory response (14-21 days) which is dependent on macrophage and T-cell dependent processes. Levels of nitrite and nitrate in plasma follows this cycling of tissue injury and inflammation with the greatest response in the secondary, chronic phase of inflammation (10-fold vs. 2-fold increase for acute phase response). Dexamethasone prevented the increase in NO production and disease status, possibly via inhibition of iNOS expression.

Chronic administration of L-NAME, a NOS inhibitor with selectivity for cNOS, has been reported to the IRA previously by the group led by M.J.S. Miller (LSU Medical Center New Orleans). In a follow-up evaluation of potential mechanisms, they provided evidence that despite expectations, NO synthesis was not prevented by chronic administration of L-NAME, rather NO production can be increased. This anomaly is the result of iNOS expression with continued administration of L-NAME. It appears that tissues respond to a reduction in NO synthesis in the basal state by expressing their back-up pathway for NO production, iNOS, in order to maintain adequate levels of NO. However, as iNOS is poorly regulated beyond translation, e.g., is not influenced by alterations in intracellular calcium, it can lead to gut inflammation in an analogous manner to more classic means of inducing iNOS expression. A word of caution would be that under basal conditions do not assume that continued administration of a NOS inhibitor, particularly cNOS specific, results in a maintained reduction in NO synthesis. Agents like aminoguanidine which are more selective for iNOS do not appear to stimulate iNOS expression in normal animals, but yet are potent anti-inflammatory agents in chronic models. Miller also presented data that suggests that peroxynitrite may contribute to the pathology associated with models of gut inflammation in which iNOS is expressed. While peroxynitrite is ephemeral at a physiological pH with a half-life of less than 1 second, it can be traced immunohistochemically with antisera to nitrotyrosine. Nitric oxide itself cannot form nitrotyrosine, but it can indirectly through nitrating agents like peroxynitrite. Nitrotyrosine immunoreactivity co-localizes with iNOS immunoreactivity in two distinct models of chronic gut inflammation induced by trinitrobenzene sulfonic acid or Freund's complete adjuvant. Furthermore, administration of the NOS inhibitor L-NAME, results in a complete suppression of nitrotyrosine immunoreactivity in addition to ameliorating the inflammatory response. In these models gene expression of iNOS parallels the time-course of inflammation and immunoreactive iNOS and nitrotyrosine, and indices of NO synthesis.

Expression of iNOS immunoreactivity and COX2 appear to be related in the chronic granulomatous model of inflammation as described by A.R. Moore. Several models of inflammation were established in rats: acute carrageenan pleurisy, Arthus reaction, and croton oil-air pouch chronic inflammation were evaluated. Immunohistochemical, biochemical and molecular (Western blot) criteria indicated that iNOS and COX2 were induced in all three models of inflammation, often in the same cell types. Data was also presented that suggested that in the air pouch model that iNOS expression may precede COX2, although the ramifications of this sequence in addition to the host of other mediators remains to be resolved. However, it was postulated that TGFβ may be a critical determinant in switching iNOS expression off prior to COX2.

The question as to the potential benefit of selective inhibitors of iNOS in inflammation was discussed at length. While it was a general consensus that iNOS appears to mediate the deleterious effects of NO it was noted that there were exceptions, with data derived from chondrocytes raised as an example. In models of arthritis the relatively poor therapeutic results obtained with aminoguanidine were discussed although aminoguanidine was noted to be very effective in gut inflammation. It is possible that some tissues are more responsive than others, or the additional actions attributed to aminoguanidine account for some of its potency in models of gut inflammation. It was also proposed that in regards to iNOS-dependent mechanisms that the role reversal displayed by NO is not merely a consequence of more of the same thing (NO), but other reactive nitrogen species like peroxynitrite, N_2O_4 and N_2O_3 that require second-order kinetics for their formation, i.e., their formation is dependent on the concentration of the substrate, or other radical species produced in the inflammatory milieu (superoxide). Considering the consequences of NO production on an arithmetical level is a gross over-simplification. As with all host defense mechanisms the issue of immunosuppression was raised as a potential complication of iNOS inhibitor therapy. However, although it was not presented, immunosuppression does not appear to be a complication of a recently developed iNOS knockout strain of mice. While this remains a concern it should not hinder drug development. Thus, while there are inconsistencies, there is a growing body of evidence supporting a pro-inflammatory role of iNOS derived NO. Selective inhibitors of this form of NOS do have excellent promise as anti-inflammatory agents with the advantage that upon restitution of health their target, iNOS, will return to its quiescent state. Time and effort will determine the accuracy of this prophecy.

POSTER DISCUSSION LIPID MEDIATORS - NEW AGENTS

G.W. DeVries* and R.S. Jacobs**
*Allergan, Inc., Irvine, CA 92715, USA
**University of California Santa Barbara, Santa Barbara, CA

A preponderance of evidence suggests that leukotrienes play a key role in a number of disease processes in which inflammation contributes significantly to the overall pathophysiology. In general, therapeutic intervention has been directed toward preventing the formation of these mediators, or designing specific antagonists to block their biological activity. Major research efforts have focused, in particular, on inhibition of 5-lipoxygenase (5-LO) and the identification of selective LTB_4 antagonists. The purpose of the poster discussion session Lipid Mediators - New Agents was to highlight new drugs which fall into these categories and to examine novel approaches for regulating arachidonic acid metabolism and, thereby, the production of lipid mediators.

R. Harris et al. (Abbott Laboratories) described the *in vivo* pharmacology of ABT-761, a second generation 5-LO inhibitor. ABT-761 was orally active in several *in vivo* models, including arachidonic acid induced mouse ear swelling (ED_{35} 6mg/kg), A23187 induced pleurisy (ED_{50} 3mg/kg) and polyacrylamide gel stimulated cell infiltration in a murine granuloma model (4 mg/kg). Administration of ABT-761 to ovalbumin challenged guinea pig led to a rapid reversal of the bronchoconstrictive response. There was much discussion regarding the potential mechanisms underlying this effect, with enzyme inhibition and very rapid turnover of mediators being postulated. It was noted, however, that once bronchoconstriction reached maximum ABT-761 was no longer able to reverse the response.

One issue regarding the development of 5-LO inhibitors has been duration of action *in vivo* and appropriate models for making this determination. Kimble et al. (Ciba Geigy) reviewed their studies of the orally active inhibitor CGS 26529. This is a highly selective 5-LO inhibitor, which was shown to have activity in the rat carrageenan-induced pleurisy and in the mouse PAF-induced mortality models. Duration of action was measured in a dog *ex vivo* model following both i.v. and oral administration. CGS 26529 (1 mg/kg) was able to inhibit A23187-stimulated LTB_4 synthesis in whole blood over a period of 24-30 hours. This was reported to be approximately 3x longer than seen with A64077 (Zileuton). SK&F 107649 was also shown to inhibit leukotriene biosynthesis *ex vivo* with a $T_{1/2} > 4$ hours (Murthy et al.). This drug was evaluated in a mouse 5% dextran sulfate mediated colitis model and shown to be active at 10 and 30 mg/kg/day orally. Although a reduction in disease severity was correlated with a reduction in LTB4 levels, the mechanism of action of SK&F 107649 was discussed in light of a concomitant decrease in TNFα levels.

The role of LTB4 as an important chemoattractant in inflammation has been well documented and is reflected in the effort to design selective LTB4 antagonists. Much less is known about the effects of peptidoleukotrienes in regulating cell infiltration. LTD4 has been reported to be a very potent chemoattractant for human eosinophils and Dutton et al. (Boots Pharmaceuticals) described their studies of murine peritoneal monocytes. Significant chemotactic activity was seen at LTD4 concentrations in the range of 0.1 - 10 nM. The pharmacologic specificity of the response was indicated by the inhibition seen in the presence of the LTD4 antagonist ICI 198,615. These results suggest that LTD4 may serve as a chemoattractant for monocytes at physiologically relevant concentrations, and that the observed anti-inflammatory effects of LTD4 antagonists may be due, in part, to their regulation of monocyte and eosinophil migration *in vivo*.

Regulation of lipid mediator synthesis has been addressed through inhibition of arachidonic acid release from phospholipids. At an earlier session, Hoffman et al. (Boehringer Ingelheim) reported differences in the kinetics of ^{3}H-arachidonic acid versus endogenous arachidonic acid release in stimulated neutrophils. These results suggested that arachidonate was released from multiple phospholipid pools, with varying potential sites for pharmacological intervention. Winkler et al. (SmithKline Beecham) described their studies of the role of CoA-independent transacylase (CoA-IT) in regulating the movement of arachidonic acid between 1-acyl and 1-alkyl phospholipid pools. Through use of the CoA-IT inhibitor SK&F 45905, they could show that blocking the movement of arachidonic acid between pools could disrupt the production of lipid mediators, such as A23187-stimulated PAF synthesis. Since these studies were done using ^{3}H-arachidonic acid, there was some discussion that the phospholipid pools being monitored may not reflect the metabolism of endogenous arachidonic acid (vis-a-vis the studies of Hoffman et al.). It is clear, however, that CoA-IT is an important enzyme in lipid mediator production and could represent a novel target for anti-inflammatory therapy.

Regulation of leukotriene production clearly can be effected by agents which directly inhibit (or activate) enzymes involved in arachidonic acid metabolism. Studies reported by Carty et al. (Pfizer, Inc.), however, suggest that changes in the intracellular ionic environment also can have significant effects on lipid mediator synthesis. Treatment of RBL cells with nigericin, which induces cytoplasmic acidification, led to a significant reduction in A23187 stimulated LTB4 production. Likewise, gramicidin inhibited LTB4 synthesis, perhaps through a change in nuclear membrane potential. Whether such a potential can be demonstrated in RBL cells and whether gramicidin freely distributes to intracellular organelles was debated. These data do suggest, however, that the 5-LO pathway can be significantly effected by regulation of intracellular ionic balance, and this approach could serve as a novel mechanism for regulating leukotriene synthesis.

In summary, work described in this poster discussion session pointed to both new pharmacologic approaches for regulating lipid mediator synthesis and novel drugs with improved anti-inflammatory activity. Harris et al. presented the *in vivo* pharmacology of a new 5-LO inhibitor ABT-761, including a rapid reversal of ovalbumin induced bronchoconstriction after intravenous injection of the drug. Two other presentations on 5-LO inhibitors dealt with pharmacokinetics. Kimble et al. discussed the unique long-acting properties of CGS 26529, and Murthy et al. discussed the effects of SK&F 107649 on LTB_4 and $TNF\alpha$ levels in a mouse model of colitis.

Dutton et al. reported on the inhibition of LTD_4 by ICI 198,615 and discussed its putative role in monocyte migration. Winkler et al. described investigations of CoA-IT in regulating arachidonic acid incorporation into phospholipid pools, while Carty et al. presented evidence that changes in intracellular pH and membrane potential may modulate mediator synthesis.

This poster discussion session was well attended, allowed for an in-depth exchange between presentors and audience, and the co-chairs felt it was clearly a worthwhile addition to the meeting format.

Subject index

208

210

AGENTS AND ACTIONS SUPPLEMENTS

Further titles in this series:

Novel Molecular Approaches to Anti-Inflammatory Therapy

Edited by **W. Pruzanski** and **P. Vadas,** *The Wellesley Hospital Research Institute, University of Toronto, Toronto, Ontario, Canada*

1995. 192 pages. Hardcover.
ISBN 3-7643-5096-2 (AAS 46)

Major advances have recently been made in our understanding of inflammatory mechanisms. These advances serve as the basis for a new generation of therapeutic agents which may potentially alter our approach to inflammatory processes and infectious diseases.

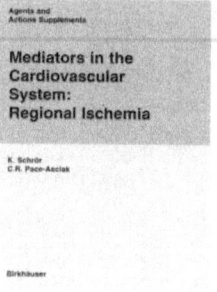

In this volume scientists of international repute describe in detail novel approaches to the study of inflammation. Topics discussed include chemokines and their role in human disease, mediation of inflammation by cyclooxygenase-2, leukocyte adhesion and the anti-inflammatory effects of leukocyte integrin blockade, anti-inflammatory lipocortin-derived peptides, and the use of anti-PECAM and other agents in the control of inflammation.

An up-to-date collection of recent research results in the field, this volume will be invaluable to pharmacologists, biochemists, biotechnologists, immunologists, rheumatologists and other clinical specialists.

Mediators in the Cardiovascular System: Regional Ischemia

Edited by **K. Schrör,** *Heinrich-Heine University, Düsseldorf, Germany*
C.R. Pace-Asciak, *Hospital for Sick Children, Toronto, ONT, Canada*

1995. 332 pages. Hardcover.
ISBN 3-7643-5130-6 (AAS 45)

The study of chemical signalling between different cell types is one of the most exciting areas in current cardiovascular research. Significant progress has been made during the last few years and a number of intercellular mediators have been structurally identified and their regulation analysed. These developments have a major impact on cardiovascular pharmacology. This includes both the molecular design of new drugs, together with an improved understanding of the actions of established compounds.

Experts of international repute address in this volume relevant aspects of recent research and emerging themes in the field of myocardial ischemia. Particular emphasis is placed upon the regulation, function and pharmacological modification of eicosanoids, nitric oxide and endothelins, with an outlook on future drug developments.

Birkhäuser Verlag • Basel • Boston • Berlin

AGENTS AND ACTIONS SUPPLEMENTS

Further titles in this series:

P.M. Brooks / R.O. Day, *University of New South Wales, Sydney, Australia /* **G.G. Graham,** *University of New South Wales, Kensington, Australia /* **K.M. Williams,** *University of New South Wales, Sydney, Australia (Eds)*

Variability in Response to Anti-Rheumatic Drugs

1993. 240 pages. Hardcover.
ISBN 3-7643-2869-X (AAS 44)

T.T. Hansel, *Sandoz Pharma Ltd., Basel, Switzerland /* **J. Morley,** *Muhmed Ltd., London, UK (Eds)*

New Drugs in Allergy and Asthma

1993. 320 pages. Hardcover.
ISBN 3-7643-2870-3 (AAS 43)

J.C. Cheronis, *Cortech, Inc., Denver, CO, USA /* **R.E. Repine,** *University of Colorado, Denver, CO, USA (Eds)*

Proteases, Protease Inhibitors and Protease-Derived Peptides

Importance in Human Pathophysiology and Therapeutics
1993. 248 pages. Hardcover.
ISBN 3-7643-2868-1 (AAS 42)

R.J. Bonney, *Bristol-Myers Squibb, Buffalo, NY, USA /* **N.S. Doherty,** *Pfizer Inc., Groton, CT, USA /* **D.W. Morgan,** *Abbott Laboratories, Abbott Park, IL, USA /* **A.F. Welton,** *Hoffman-La-Roche Inc., Nutley, NJ, USA (Eds)*

Inflammatory Disease Therapy: Preclinical and Clinical Developments

1993. 209 pages. Hardcover.
ISBN 3-7643-2859-2 (AAS 41)

M.H. Schöni, *Alpine Kinderklinik, Davos, Switzerland /* **R. Kraemer,** *Inselspital, Bern, Switzerland (Eds)*

Update on Childhood Asthma

1993. 222 pages. Hardcover.
ISBN 3-7643-2867-3 (AAS 40)

W.B. van den Berg / P.M. van der Kraan / P.L.E.M. van Lent, *Dept. of Rheumatology, University Hospital, Nijmegen, The Netherlands (Eds)*

Joint Destruction in Arthritis and Osteoarthritis

1993. 276 pages. Hardcover.
ISBN 3-7643-2773-1 (AAS 39)

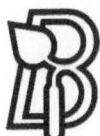

Birkhäuser Verlag • Basel • Boston • Berlin

AGENTS AND ACTIONS SUPPLEMENTS

Further titles in this series:

H. Fritz, W. Müller-Esterl,
M. Jochum, A. Roscher, K. Luppertz
(Vol. 38/I);
G. Bönner, H. Fritz, Th. Unger,
A. Roscher, K. Luppertz (Vol. 38/II);
G. Bönner, H. Fritz, B. Schoelkens,
G. Dietze, K. Luppertz (Vol. 38/III)

Recent Progress on Kinins

1992. 1750 pages. Hardcover.
ISBN 3-7643-2816-9 (AAS 38)

H. F. Sinzinger / K. Schrör (Eds)

Prostaglandins in the Cardiovascular System

1992. 392 pages. Hardcover.
ISBN 3-7643-2701-4 (AAS 37)

A.M. Rothschild (Ed.)

Contributions to Autacoid Pharmacology

1992. 296 pages. Hardcover.
ISBN 3-7643-2617-4 (AAS 36)

N.R. Ackerman / R. J. Bonney /
A.F. Welton (Eds)

Progress in Inflammation Research and Therapy

1991. XVI + 192 pages. Hardcover.
ISBN 3-7643-2529-1 (AAS 35)

G.P. Anderson / I.D. Chapman /
J. Morley (Eds)

New Drugs for Asthma Therapy

1991.560 pages. Hardcover.
ISBN 3-7643-2505-4 (AAS 34)

H. Timmermann / H. van der Goot
(Eds)

New Perspectives in Histamine Research

1991. 434 pages. Hardcover.
ISBN 3-7643-2507-0 (AAS 33)

M.J. Parnham / M.A. Bray /
W.B. van den Berg (Eds)

Drugs in Inflammation

1991. 264 pages. Hardcover.
ISBN 3-7643-2504-6 (AAS 32)

F. Nijkamp / F. Engels /
P.A.J. Henricks /
A.J.M. van Oosterhout (Eds)

Mediators in Airway Hyperreactivity

1990. 295 pages. Hardcover.
ISBN 3-7643-2513-5 (AAS 31)

C. Persson / R. Brettsand / L. Laitinen
P. Venge (Eds)

Inflammatory Indices in Chronic Bronchitis

1990. 294 pages. Hardcover
ISBN 3-7643-2370-1(AAS 30)

Birkhäuser Verlag • Basel • Boston • Berlin